SPELT

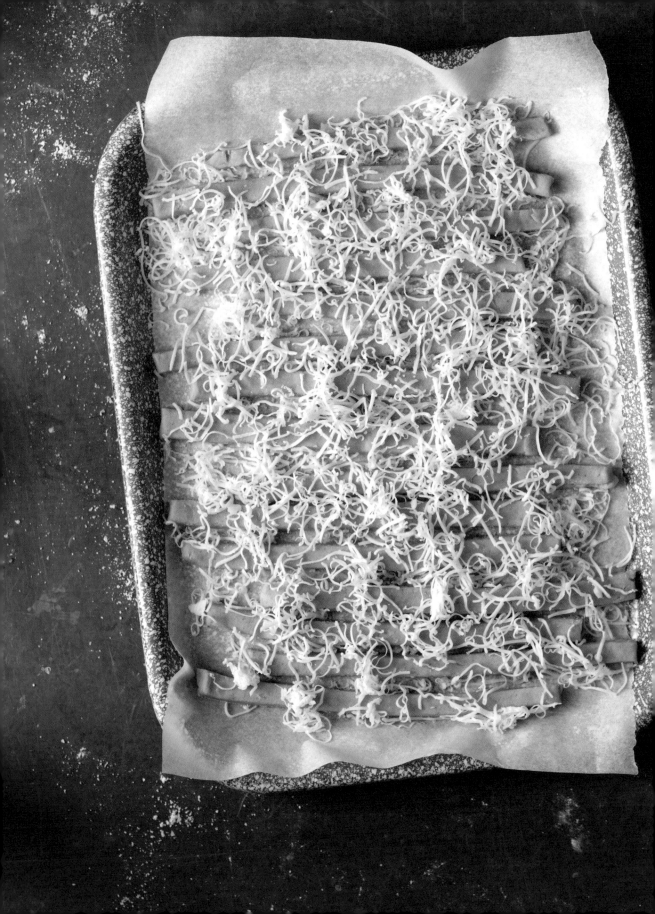

SPELT

CAKES, COOKIES, BREADS & MEALS FROM THE GOOD GRAIN

ROGER SAUL

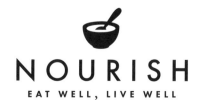

NOURISH
EAT WELL, LIVE WELL

To my soulmate, Monty

Spelt
Roger Saul

First published in the United Kingdom and Ireland in
2015 by Nourish, an imprint of Watkins Media Limited
19 Cecil Court
London WC2N 4HE

enquiries@nourishbooks.com

Publisher: Grace Cheetham
Managing Editor: Rebecca Woods
Editor: Wendy Hobson
Art Direction and Design: Georgina Hewitt
Production: Uzma Taj
Commissioned Photography: Lara Holmes
(except pages 6, 20–1, 44–5, 66–7, 94–5, 122–3,
152–3: Neil White, and page 7: Tyson Sadlo)
Food Stylists: Signe Johansen and Aya Nishimura
Prop Stylist: Wei Tang
Nutritional Consultants: Amanda Hamilton and
Jessica Andersson

A CIP record for this book is available from the British
Library

ISBN: 978-1-84899-229-0

10 9 8 7 6 5 4 3 2 1

Typeset in Garamond
Colour reproduction by PDQ, UK
Printed in China

Publisher's note:
While every care has been taken in compiling the recipes
for this book, Watkins Media Limited, or any other
persons who have been involved in working on this publi-
cation, cannot accept responsibility for any errors or omis-
sions, inadvertent or not, that may be found in the recipes
or text, nor for any problems that may arise as a result
of preparing one of these recipes. If you are pregnant or
breastfeeding or have any special dietary requirements or
medical conditions, it is advisable to consult a medical
professional before following any of the recipes contained
in this book. Spelt contains gluten and is not suitable for
coeliacs or anyone allergic/intolerant to gluten.

Notes on the recipes:
Unless otherwise stated:
Use organic produce, wherever possible
Use medium eggs, fruit and vegetables
Use fresh ingredients, including herbs and chillies
Use unwaxed lemons
Do not mix metric and imperial measurements
1 tsp = 5ml 1 tbsp = 15ml 1 cup = 250ml

nourishbooks.com

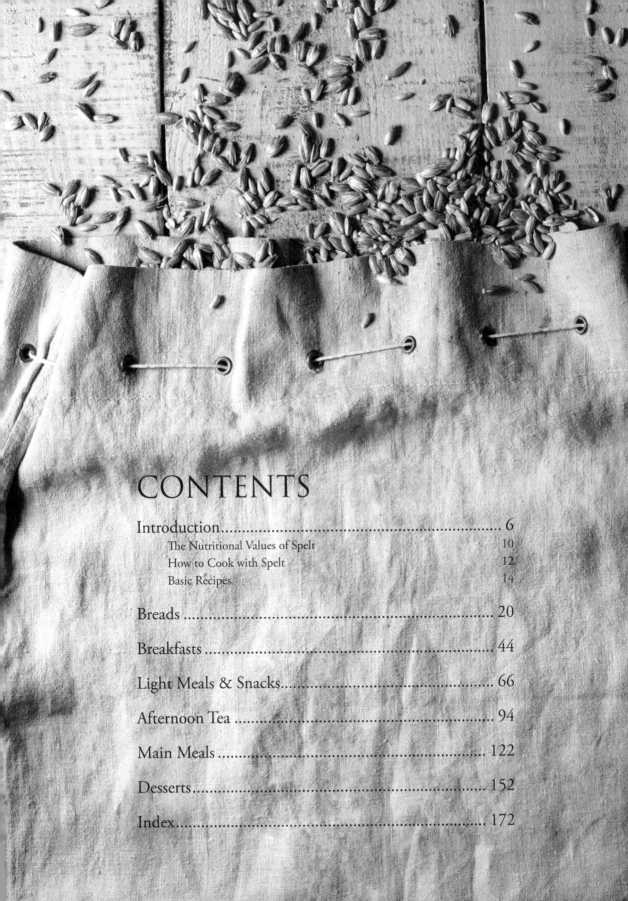

CONTENTS

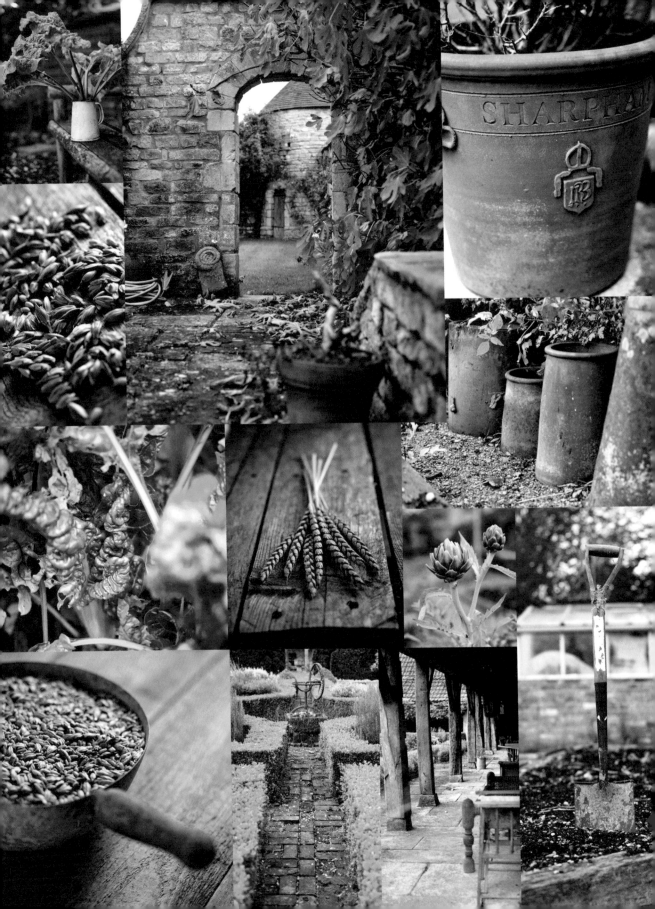

INTRODUCTION

'Why don't you grow spelt?' suggested my sister Rosemary as we sat in the kitchen of Sharpham Park. It was 2003, and my wife Monty and I had just bought the farmland around our lovely old abbots' house, where we had lived for 26 years, and were trying to decide what we should grow.

Rosemary's doctor had advised spelt as a gentle but nourishing alternative to conventional wheat. She was undergoing cancer treatment at the time and wanted to find foods that would boost her health and support her fragile body during treatment. What she said made me curious, and I set about researching the grain on the internet.

Spelt, I discovered, has ancient beginnings and potentially significant health benefits. It was virtually unheard of at the time, and my visits to health-food stores turned up small, dense and dull-tasting loaves on the top shelf, and some only slightly more tasty crackers. There were no growers in the UK at the time, so I set out to find and buy seed in France, Italy and Germany (my trading languages coming in handy from my days establishing and running the Mulberry designer brand!). In French, spelt is called *l'epeautre*, in Italian, *farro* and to the Germans, it is known as *dinkel*.

I found out that spelt had been grown for some 4,000 years in the area that we live in, since the Bronze and Iron Ages. Carbonized grains of spelt had been found in food remains in the Glastonbury Lake Village excavations. Researching Sharpham Park's history, I learnt that it had a rich and varied farming background, stretching back centuries. The land is first mentioned in AD 978 when King Edwig of Wessex gave it to the thegn Aetholwold. It then passed in and out of the hands of the abbots of Glastonbury for the next 500 years. By 1300 it had been enclosed as a deer park by the abbots, land that would have provided every kind of food for the monks' table, with tenant farmers growing a variety of different crops, which would, without doubt, have included spelt.

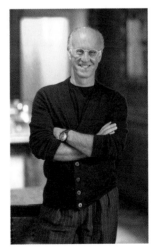

The business part of my brain knew that to create a whole new 'Sharpham Park' brand I would need a certain something to be the 'hero' product. Instinctively, I knew I had found it. You might ask, why would someone whose background was in fashion design and marketing even contemplate farming? Well, as a small boy I would stay on my grandparents' Suffolk farm during the long summer holidays, and whether I was helping to feed the pigs or riding the combine harvester, I was always in seventh heaven. To have a farm of my own was both thrilling and terrifying in equal measure. But also, in a strange way, it felt like coming home.

Our first steps in organic farming were both educational and an eye-opener. We were told by our Soil Association adviser that it would be wise to convert half our landholding to organic status

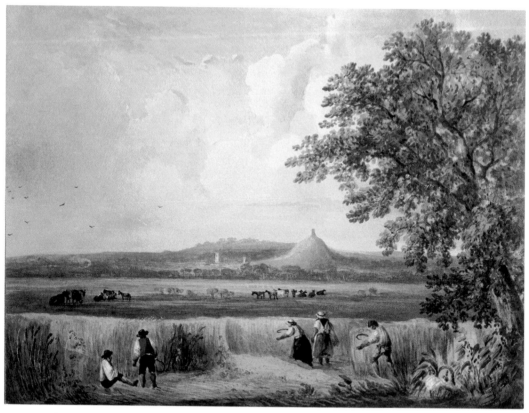

Above: Painting of Sharpham Park and Glastonbury Tor, Rev. W.W. Wheatley, 1843

first, so we could get used to the process. The first lesson was salutary. We watched as our lovely team sprayed the conventional wheat crops with fertilizer, pesticides, weedkillers and even growth inhibitors so that the wheat would grow to exactly 39cm/15½in for the ease of the combine harvester. These fields looked impressive. Our organic spelt, by contrast, looked a bedraggled mess, full of weeds, nettles and flowers. I started to think, what have I done? But then the spelt began to grow through, and went on growing until it was 1.5m/5ft tall. Since then, we've never looked back.

That year of farming both conventionally and organically was the best thing we ever did. It helped us to understand that the efficient bug-killing regimes that have their place in mass food production (but are banned in organic growing) can and do destroy the insect lifecycle so vital not only to natural bug control but also to the birds and wildlife dependent on them for food. These sprays break down natural immune systems and have done untold damage in destroying the micro-organisms in our soils. We felt that it was time to change all that, and we embarked upon a cycle of organic crop rotation, a system that is used to restore the essential nitrogen, potassium and other minerals in the soil so that crop yields are kept naturally high.

In our first spelt trial, we grew three different types, and found that a hardy old German variety was the best for our soil type and climate. Dehusking the grain presented a real challenge, as one of spelt's natural features is its extra-strong outer husk. Luckily, we found a wonderful local watermill, and the owners kindly agreed to have a set of millstones put back into production, especially for our organic spelt.

Finally, when we had our first flour all bagged up, we told the story to Tamasin Day-Lewis, food writer for the *Daily Telegraph*. She wrote our very first press story about the rebirth of spelt. We were inundated with readers' enquiries. Each person had their own tale to tell, often of sensitivity to ordinary wheat, and were desperate to know where they could buy our spelt.

We went on to build our own mill, the only one in the world milling solely stone-ground organic spelt, which was kindly opened by Sophie, Countess of Wessex, in June 2007.

SO WHAT IS SPELT?

Spelt is a member of the grain family, but it has certain properties that make it quite different from wheat, barley, oats or rye. It is a hybrid of emmer wheat and goat grass, and has a distinctive, nutty flavour. There is plenty of evidence that spelt was cultivated by early civilizations, such as in Mesopotamia in the Middle East, around 9,000 years ago. In Britain it is first known to have existed as a main crop in 2000 BCE. Later, it came to be known as the Roman army's marching grain. According to legend, warriors in the area now known as Germany ate spelt before going into battle. The Roman legionaries who fought them were so impressed that they added spelt to their diets, too. They would cover vast distances, transporting this vital fuel, sustained by its slow-release energy. Known as *farrum*, it was used to create a leavened bread that consisted of spelt flour, olive oil, salt, yeast, water and honey.

With the major migrations from Europe to America in the late 1800s, spelt moved with them, and by 1910 more than 600,000 acres of spelt were harvested annually. By the 1970s, however, production in the USA had almost died out with the advent of modern farming techniques and the hybridization of wheat, which meant more efficient harvests. The same trend happened in Europe – old-fashioned grains like spelt, which has a husk that protects it from the ravages of both insect and weather, fell out of fashion. The husk is difficult to remove and, once it has been, the yield is 40 per cent lower than wheat. Modern wheat has been bred to lose its husk during harvesting.

The husk, however, has various valuable attributes. It protects and shields the grain from disease-carrying insects, eliminating the need for toxic pesticides, and is essential for germination. We store our spelt with its husk on and it will last for years if stored at the right temperature. We separate it from the kernel before we stone-mill the grain, thus preserving the grain's freshness as well as its nutrients.

THE NUTRITIONAL VALUES OF SPELT

I always worry that harping on about what is 'good for you' might turn many food-lovers off, and make them suspicious that they're going to be in for something unpalatable. With spelt, nothing could be further from the truth. Unlike some of the rather bland alternative grains on the health-food store shelf, spelt tastes like a nuttier version of fluffy wheat. And yes, it's good for you, too!

Spelt is truly a wholegrain, in contrast to so many of the pretenders on the shelves these days. Unlike much wheat, where the nutritional benefits of bran and germ are largely removed during milling, the good stuff in spelt is found in the inner kernel of the grain, and so survives the milling process unscathed.

It has become a popular cereal for those following a lower-carb lifestyle as spelt bread contains almost 50 per cent more protein than wheat-based bread. It is also popular with many who suffer from an intolerance to modern wheat varieties. (It must, however, be noted that spelt is not gluten free, and is therefore not suitable for coeliacs or anyone allergic/intolerant to gluten.) So what is it about spelt that makes people feel good?

IT BEATS THE BLOAT
Everyday bloating, usually caused by wind or water retention, can make you feel self-conscious and your clothes tight and uncomfortable. Once you've ruled out a serious gastrointestinal condition or a food intolerance or allergy as the cause, making the choice of spelt rather than wheat can help you banish the bloat. Spelt is low in a group of short-chain carbohydrates named FODMAPs (here comes a mouthful!) – Fermentable Oligosaccharides Disaccharides, Monosaccharides and Polyols – which are poorly absorbed in the small intestine and rapidly ferment, causing symptoms of wind and bloating.

It seems that sensitive digestive systems find spelt is more easily tolerated than those varieties of modern wheat that have been bred to contain a high gluten content for the production of high-volume baked goods. This could be because spelt has a more fragile gluten structure (shorter and more brittle), which is easier to digest as it is more water soluble than modern wheat.

IT'S HIGH IN FIBRE
Spelt's high fibre content not only makes it easier to digest the gluten, but it is important for lowering cholesterol levels in the blood, too. In addition, foods with a high fibre content pass through the gut more quickly, and research shows that faster transit time (how long it takes for food to travel through the digestive tract) is an important factor in bowel cancer prevention.

IT PROVIDES SLOW-RELEASE ENERGY

The structure of the long chain molecules in the spelt grain are important because they help your body digest the grain slowly. Spelt also has a lower GI ('glycaemic index': the effect that different foods have on blood glucose levels) than many grains. Many people are sensibly learning to avoid high-GI carbs found in refined foods, which cause glucose 'spikes' to hit your bloodstream and can lead to all kinds of health problems, including type-2 diabetes. It is thought that spelt may help improve insulin sensitivity, so that your body needs lower levels of the hormone to balance blood glucose levels.

IT'S A NATURAL VITAMIN AND MINERAL SOURCE

Spelt grain is a good source of nutrients; it's high in B vitamins, which help to break down and release energy from food, keep nerves and muscle tissue healthy as well as aid skin, digestive system and eye health. It contains vitamin E, which helps to protect the cells from the damaging effects of free radicals. It is rich in the mineral magnesium, which is important for activating muscles and nerves and creating energy in the body. Spelt also contains potassium and iron. Potassium is vital to help nerves and muscles communicate, while iron provides oxygen to blood cells. Finally, it is rich in manganese, which plays an important role in the digestion and utilisation of food, normal bone structure and the functioning of the central nervous system.

IT'S GOOD FOR YOUR HEART, BLOOD AND BONES

Spelt is an excellent source of phytoestrogens and lignans. Phytoestrogens are plant compounds that scientists believe may help blood cholesterol levels, blood vessel elasticity, bone metabolism and many other vital cellular metabolic processes. Research on lignans has also thrown up some interesting results for spelt-lovers. It is thought that these phytonutrients may influence the development of tumours in hormone-related cancers, slowing down their growth, as well as having a positive effect on cardiovascular health. Spelt is also thought to help moderate the symptoms of menopause and osteoporosis.

IT'S A HEALTHY SOURCE OF PROTEIN

The protein in the spelt we produce at Sharpham has historically made up between 11 and 15 per cent of the grain, depending on the growing season and weather conditions. These proteins contain all of the nine essential amino acids needed by the human body (called 'essential' because the body cannot manufacture them on its own).

IT MIGHT EVEN MAKE YOU HAPPIER TOO!

Recently, scientists have confirmed what naturopaths have been suggesting for years – that your gut 'brain', the enteric nervous system, is innately linked to your immune system, and that your digestive health can have a direct effect on your emotional state. Patients suffering from irritable bowel syndrome (IBS) or other digestive disorders can also suffer from anxiety and depression. I am a firm believer that keeping your tummy happy can help keep you happy, too, and as spelt can aid with digestion and bloating, it could be the perfect prescription.

HOW TO COOK WITH SPELT

Spelt really is a cook's best friend. It's great for making bread and cakes, and it can also make pastry and biscuits with a wonderful, crisp texture. The nutty flavour of spelt makes everything taste good, and the flour behaves in much the same way as wheat, if not better, so you don't really have to learn any new techniques.

I think it's always best to think of recipes as a guide, rather than strict instructions to be rigidly adhered to, so it's important to practice using spelt in a variety of ways. It won't take long for you to get used to using it – and once you do, you'll never look back.

BREAD

As there is generally a higher protein content and a more delicate gluten structure in spelt flour, you don't need to knead it for as long as when making wheat bread Remember, though, that it is more hygroscopic than refined flour, which means the dough will require a little more liquid, as you work the ingredients together, to prevent it from drying out. If your bread dough is feeling a little dry when you're kneading, make sure you don't just push on; instead, add more liquid. As bakers will tell you, the wetter the dough, the better the bread will be. Never shy away from adding more water, milk or other appropriate liquid to keep the dough soft and supple. A dough that is dry and tough after 10 minutes of kneading isn't going to improve after proving and baking.

Lievito Bakery, who make the flatbreads for our restaurant at Kilver Court in Somerset, have some great advice when it comes to making bread with spelt:

- Bake it in a tin or basket. The gluten structure in spelt is different to that in wheat flour and it's the network of fine gluten strands that gives the dough its structure, so a spelt loaf will benefit from being supported as it cooks.

- Spelt dough can be quite dense. To make it softer, add a tablespoon of clear honey to give a pliable texture and to bring out the flavour.

- To loosen the bread, add some fat – a little unsalted butter will do the job, and it's better than oil.

PASTRY

Due to our spelt flour being stoneground, not highly refined or bleached in the way of some modern wheat varieties and brands, the pastries in this book may not look quite as pale and golden blonde as you might expect, but I think the nutty flavour will be much more delicious. It's worth pointing out that the gluten in spelt behaves differently from the gluten in wheat and doesn't over-develop, which makes it easy to work with and results in reliably crumbly, crisp pastries and biscuits.

There are some useful cook's tricks that can keep pastry doughs extra-crisp when you bake them. For example, chilling the dough in a fridge or freezer before rolling it out really helps to keep both the shape and the texture of the pastry when baked. If you're working in a warm kitchen, using a marble slab can also help in keeping the dough chilled when rolling out. If the shaped pastry starts to soften or sweat a little, then simply chill it again before you bake it.

CAKES AND COOKIES

Cakes such as Summer Raspberry Cake (see page 108) are really easy to make with spelt flour, for the same reason spelt makes such good pastries and biscuits. The flour doesn't over-develop when added to liquid so you can fold it into a mixture without worrying about a tough, chewy result like you could potentially get with plain wheat flour. Cookies are given an extra wholesome flavour with spelt due to its nutty taste, and not only will they taste delicious but they'll be that little bit more nutritious too. Why not give Ginger and Honey Cookies (see page 97) a try next time you crave something sweet?

STEWS, SALADS & RISOTTOS

As you'll see, spelt is more than just milled into flour. It can also be pearled, flaked and turned into couscous. In fact, anything wheat can do, I like to think spelt can do better. At Sharpham Park we pearl our grain between five rotating stones to remove the outer layer of bran. It is delicious in a risotto, or 'Speltotto' (see pages 136–137), and the polished grain plumps up to twice its original size as it absorbs the water, flavoured with all of the ingredients. Pearled spelt has all the nutty, wholesome flavour you would expect of the whole grain, but it takes a mere 20 minutes to cook. We also love using it in salads, soups and stews – simply follow the directions on the pearled spelt packet and treat it as an alternative to brown rice, barley or other trendy grains such as quinoa.

MUESLI & PORRIDGE

Finally, we would be remiss if we didn't mention satisfying spelt breakfasts. Prepare Monty's Muesli (see page 48) and enjoy a spring and summertime version topped with fresh berries. Or try Swiss-Style Bircher Muesli (see page 48), a cold muesli that requires overnight soaking. This is considered a highly digestible way of eating grains, so once the days get longer and the temperature rises, don't forego your daily bowl. Simply soak the spelt grains, then enjoy them the next day with some fruit, nuts and seeds of your choice. As autumn and winter approach, few things beat a bowl of piping-hot Porridge (see page 49), topped with home-made jam, or a drizzle of honey. Spelt porridge flakes behave in much the same way as oats and make a fantastic start in the morning – charging your batteries for the day ahead.

BASIC RECIPES

The basic recipes I have included here are your stalwarts to make any number of delicious things. Shortcrust Pastry provides you with the perfect base for tarts and quiches. Rough Puff Pastry is your route to endless pies, and don't forget vol au vents! Spelt Pasta is in a world of its own, and once you get into experimenting with it, family and friends won't leave you alone! Refined white spelt flour just makes for a delicious pasta base. Finally, I have included a recipe for a basic Sourdough Starter as, for me, spelt sourdough is the king of all breads.

Because of its lower gluten content, spelt flour makes excellent pastry – perfectly crisp and with a slightly nutty flavour. This is the basic pastry recipe that we use for any number of delicious tarts, savoury or sweet, such as Broccoli & Courgette Quiche (see page 76) and Lemon Tart (see page 161).

SHORTCRUST PASTRY

MAKES enough to line a 23cm/9in tart tin
PREPARATION TIME: 15 minutes, plus 1 hour chilling COOKING TIME: 15 minutes

Put the flour in a large bowl, then rub in the cold butter, using your fingertips, until the mixture resembles fine breadcrumbs. Stir in the caster sugar, then the egg, then gradually add about 2 tablespoons cold water, a drop at a time, to bind everything to a smooth dough. Cover the dough with cling film and chill in the fridge for about 1 hour to relax the dough.

When you're ready to roll out the pastry, preheat the oven to 180°C/350°F/Gas 4 and grease a tart tin suitable for the recipe.

To bake blind, turn the dough out onto a lightly floured work surface and roll out to 5mm/¼in thick. Use to line the prepared tart tin and trim the edges. Line the pastry case with a piece of baking paper and cover with baking beans. Bake for 10 minutes, then remove the paper and baking beans and bake for a further 5 minutes until just golden.

220g/7¾oz/1¾ cups white or wholegrain spelt flour, plus extra for dusting.......................................
115g/4oz cold salted butter, cubed .....
1 tbsp golden caster sugar..................
1 egg, beaten ....

Rough puff pastry is great for savoury pies, with its crumbly texture, golden colour and the lovely glaze you can give it with just a little beaten egg. It does take a little time and a bit of effort, but it is very rewarding.

ROUGH PUFF PASTRY

MAKES enough to line a 23cm/9in tart tin
PREPARATION TIME: 15 minutes, plus 1 hour chilling COOKING TIME: 15 minutes

Mix together the flour, butter and salt in a large bowl, then gradually start to add 275ml/9 ½ fl oz/1 cup plus 1 tablespoon cold water and knead very gently until just incorporated. The dough should not be smooth. Shape the dough into a rectangle about 2cm/½in thick, wrap in cling film and chill in the fridge for 20 minutes to relax the pastry.

When rested, take the pastry from the fridge and roll out in one direction on a lightly floured work surface into a long rectangle. Fold the bottom up two-thirds and the top down one-third to meet the fold. Fold over exactly in half, as if you were closing a book. Give the dough a 90-degree turn and repeat the process. Wrap in cling film and rest in the fridge for 20 more minutes to relax the pastry, then repeat the whole process twice more, or until there are no longer any streaks of butter in the pastry. Chill the pastry for a final 20 minutes, then roll it out into a sheet or circle, or any other appropriate shape. Keep the trimmings for other pastry items or for pie decorations.

500g/1lb 2oz/4 cups white
    spelt flour, plus extra for dusting......
500g/1lb 2oz cold unsalted butter,
    finely diced ....
2 tsp sea salt ....

Spelt pasta is one of my favourite dishes. The combination of the unique texture with that slightly nutty flavour makes it extra special. Hopefully this will persuade you to never buy that supermarket packet ever again! We have used refined white spelt flour here, but you can use wholegrain instead, if you prefer, which gives a much heavier, grainier pasta. Dusting with semolina stops the strands from sticking together and allows you to roll it out thinly. Don't forget to have a broomstick handy to hang the pasta on to dry!

PASTA

MAKES 600g/1lb 5oz
PREPARATION TIME: 30 minutes, plus 30 minutes chilling and rolling out

Put the flour on a clean work surface and make a well in the centre. Pour the beaten eggs into this well and start bringing the flour and eggs together. Keep mixing until the ingredients are blended into a rough dough.

Transfer the dough to a lightly floured work surface and knead by turning, stretching and folding for 5–10 minutes until you have a soft, pliable dough. Shape the dough into a flat disc and wrap well with cling film, then chill in the fridge for 30 minutes to relax the dough.

Remove it from the fridge and roll out and cut to whichever shape you wish, scattering a little semolina over the cut pasta to keep the pieces from sticking together. If you are making long pasta, hang the strands over a clean broom handle to dry out or use two wire racks resting against each other to form a triangle.

500g/1lb 2oz/4 cups white spelt flour, plus extra for dusting ....
5 eggs, lightly beaten ....
1 handful of semolina to separate the pasta strands ....

There is a lot of angst about creating a 'mother' – a sourdough starter – and sustaining her, but it is actually incredibly simple. Once your starter is working, you can gradually add to it and it will improve in flavour. Use this starter to make a classic Sourdough Bread (see page 24), or the festive Sourdough Stollen (see page 37) at Christmas.

SOURDOUGH STARTER

MAKES about 600g/1lb 5oz starter
PREPARATION TIME: 5 days

Put 150ml/5fl oz/⅔ cup lukewarm water in a 500ml/17fl oz/2 cup glass preserving jar with the Day 1 ingredients, stir well, then cover and leave at room temperature for 24 hours.

Add the Day 2 ingredients and 55ml/2fl oz/4 tablespoons lukewarm water, stir well, cover and leave again at room temperature for 24 hours.

The mixture will start to change colour, the raisins will start to dissolve and there will be a bubble or two on the surface. Add the Day 3 ingredients with 100ml/3½fl oz/scant ½ cup lukewarm water, stir well, cover and leave as before for 24 hours.

You should be able to sniff the fermentation. Throw away three-quarters of the mixture and add 100ml/3½fl oz/scant ½ cup lukewarm water. Strain to remove the raisins, then return the liquid to the preserving jar. Add the Day 4 flour, mix well, cover and leave as before for 24 hours.

Repeat on Day 5, when you'll notice an acidic tang to the mix.

On Day 6, the mixture should be bubbling and ready to use.

Each time you remove some of the mother, simply replace it with the same quantity of flour and water. As time goes on, the mother will become more acidic and take on more flavour and character.

DAY 1
2 tsp wholegrain spelt flour ....
2 tsp white spelt flour ....
2 tsp raisins ....
2 tsp natural bio yogurt ....
DAY 2
2 tsp wholegrain spelt flour ....
2 tsp white spelt flour ....
DAY 3
4 tsp wholegrain spelt flour ....
4 tsp white spelt flour ....
DAY 4
125g/4½oz/1 cup white spelt flour .....
DAY 5
125g/4½oz/1 cup white spelt flour .....

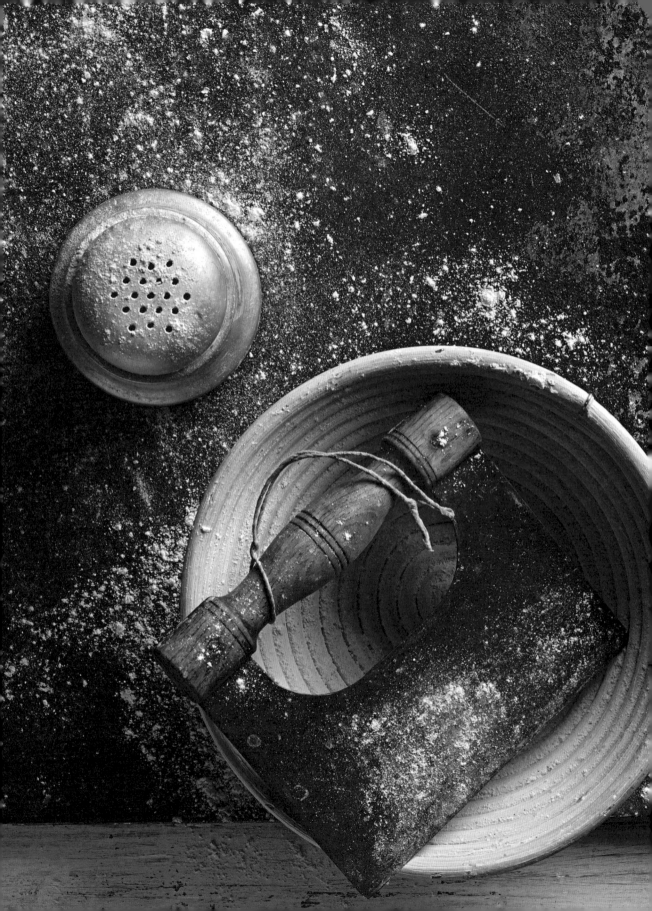

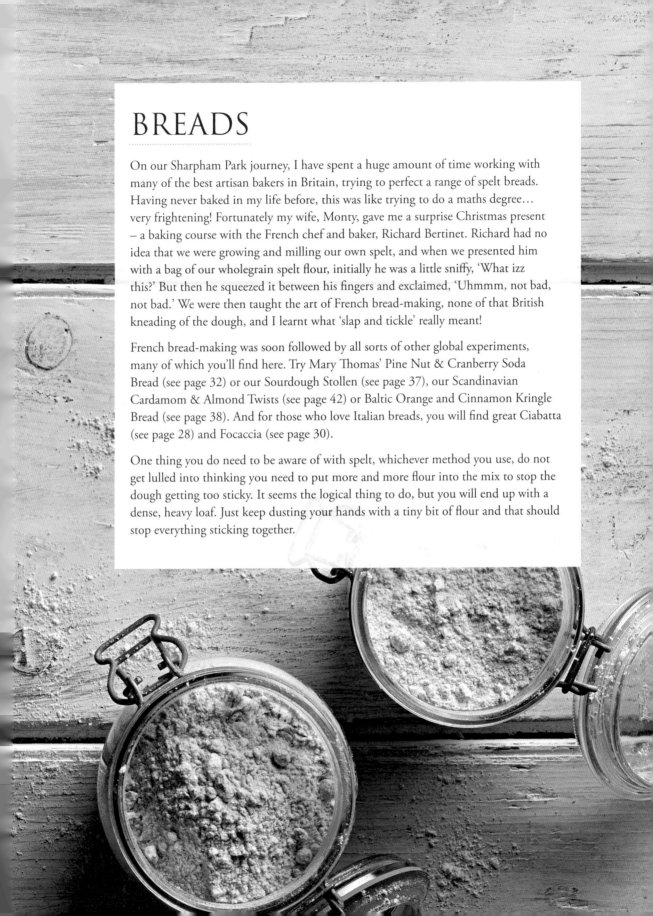

BREADS

On our Sharpham Park journey, I have spent a huge amount of time working with many of the best artisan bakers in Britain, trying to perfect a range of spelt breads. Having never baked in my life before, this was like trying to do a maths degree… very frightening! Fortunately my wife, Monty, gave me a surprise Christmas present – a baking course with the French chef and baker, Richard Bertinet. Richard had no idea that we were growing and milling our own spelt, and when we presented him with a bag of our wholegrain spelt flour, initially he was a little sniffy, 'What izz this?' But then he squeezed it between his fingers and exclaimed, 'Uhmmm, not bad, not bad.' We were then taught the art of French bread-making, none of that British kneading of the dough, and I learnt what 'slap and tickle' really meant!

French bread-making was soon followed by all sorts of other global experiments, many of which you'll find here. Try Mary Thomas' Pine Nut & Cranberry Soda Bread (see page 32) or our Sourdough Stollen (see page 37), our Scandinavian Cardamom & Almond Twists (see page 42) or Baltic Orange and Cinnamon Kringle Bread (see page 38). And for those who love Italian breads, you will find great Ciabatta (see page 28) and Focaccia (see page 30).

One thing you do need to be aware of with spelt, whichever method you use, do not get lulled into thinking you need to put more and more flour into the mix to stop the dough getting too sticky. It seems the logical thing to do, but you will end up with a dense, heavy loaf. Just keep dusting your hands with a tiny bit of flour and that should stop everything sticking together.

SHARPHAM PARK FARMHOUSE LOAF

MAKES 2 x 450g/1lb loaves
PREPARATION TIME: 30 minutes, plus 2½ hours rising COOKING TIME: 50 minutes

Lightly oil a large bowl and two 450g/1lb loaf tins. In a small bowl, dissolve the yeast in 290ml/10fl oz/1 cup plus 2 tablespoons lukewarm water. Put the flour and salt in another large bowl and make a well in the centre. Add the yeast mixture, butter and honey and mix together, using a wooden spoon, to a rough dough.

Turn the dough out onto a lightly floured work surface and knead for 5–8 minutes until the dough is smooth and elastic and springs back when poked. Transfer the kneaded dough to the prepared bowl, cover with a clean, damp tea towel and leave to rise in a warm place for 1 hour, or until doubled in size.

Turn the dough out onto a lightly floured work surface. Knock the air out of the dough by punching it with your fist and expel the gas by pressing down onto the dough, then folding it back on itself like an envelope. Return the dough to the bowl, cover again and leave in a warm place for a further 30 minutes, or until it has doubled in size again and no longer springs back when poked.

On a floured work surface, divide the dough in half and shape each piece into a ball. Cover with a clean, damp tea towel and leave to rest for a further 10 minutes.

Shape the dough into blocks and put in the prepared loaf tins. Cover again and leave in a warm place for 50–60 minutes until almost doubled in size.

Preheat the oven to 210°C/410°F/Gas 6–7.

Dust the loaves with a little spelt flour or spelt porridge flakes, if using. Turn the oven down to 190°C/375°F/Gas 5 and bake for 40–50 minutes until golden on top and hollow-sounding when tapped. If you prefer a crustier loaf, bake for 35 minutes, take the loaves out of the tins, then return them to the oven for the last 10–15 minutes of the baking time, sitting them directly on the middle oven shelf. Transfer to a wire rack to cool.

a little oil, for greasing ....
10g/⅓oz/1 tbsp fresh yeast, crumbled, or 4g/⅛oz/1 tsp fast-action dried yeast ....
470g/1lb 1oz/3¾ cups white spelt flour, plus extra for dusting ....
2 tsp sea salt ....
1 tbsp unsalted butter, softened ....
2 tsp clear honey ....
2 tsp spelt porridge flakes (optional) ...

COOKS' TIP
Warm proving is fine and will produce a good result for breads generally, but for more in-depth and complex flavours, you could try cold proving. For example, you could make a dough in the morning, leave it in a cool place all day, then finish and bake it in the evening, allowing a cold prove of some 6–8 hours. Artisan bread-making is usually done over 2–3 days of 'fermentation', especially with sourdough.

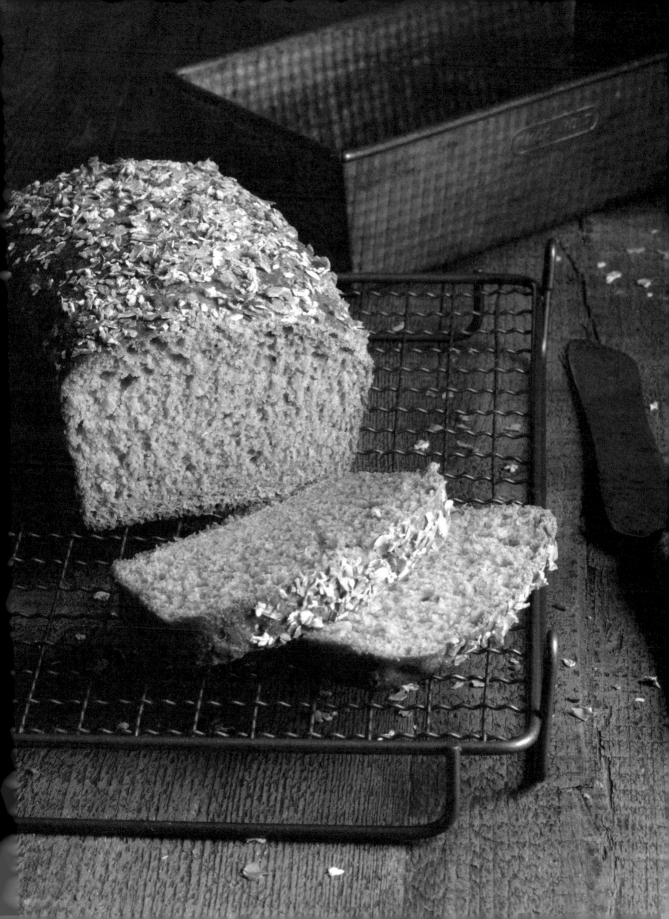

This nutritious, nutty wholemeal loaf is full of grains and seeds. It is chewy and rustic, the way really good bread should be. If you leave the dough to ferment overnight in the fridge, you only need half the quantity of yeast, as the yeast multiplies over the longer proving time. This produces an even more delicious and complex-flavoured loaf. It also makes the best toast because the lightly toasted seeds and spelt combine to give a great taste. You can use equal quantities of wholegrain and white spelt flour, if you prefer.

SEEDED LOAF

MAKES 900g/2lb loaf
PREPARATION TIME: 30 minutes, plus 1¼ hours rising COOKING TIME: 1¼ hours

Lightly oil a large bowl and a 900g/2lb loaf tin. Cook the pearled spelt in boiling water for 20 minutes, or until tender, following the packet instructions. Drain and leave to cool slightly.

Sift the flour into another large bowl and make a well in the centre. Add 350ml/12fl oz/scant 1½ cups lukewarm water, the oil, yeast, sugar, if using, treacle, salt and cooked pearled spelt, if using, and mix together, using a wooden spoon, to a rough dough.

Turn the dough out onto a lightly floured work surface and knead for 5–8 minutes until the dough is smooth and elastic and springs back when poked. Transfer the kneaded dough to the prepared bowl, cover with a clean, damp tea towel and leave to rise in a warm place for 45 minutes, or until doubled in size.

Turn the dough out onto a lightly floured work surface and roll out to 1cm/½in thick. Reserve 1 tablespoon of the mixed seeds, then sprinkle the remainder over the dough. Fold the dough to incorporate the seeds, then shape into a rectangular block and put in the prepared loaf tin. Cover again and leave to rise in a warm place for a further 30 minutes until the dough has doubled in size and no longer springs back when poked.

Preheat the oven to 220°C/425°F/Gas 7. When you're ready to bake the loaf, beat the egg with 2 tablespoons water to make an egg wash, then brush over the top of the loaf and sprinkle with the reserved seeds and the spelt porridge flakes. Splash a little water in the bottom of the oven to create steam to help the bread to rise. Bake just above the centre for 10–15 minutes, then turn the oven down to 190°C/375°F/Gas 5 and bake for a further 30–40 minutes, or until the bread is well risen, firm and hollow-sounding when tapped. Transfer to a wire rack to cool.

1 tbsp sunflower oil, plus extra for greasing ....
55g/2oz/heaped ¼ cup pearled spelt...
500g/1lb 2oz/4 cups wholegrain spelt flour ....
10g/⅓oz/1 tbsp fresh yeast, crumbled, or 4g/⅛oz/1 tsp fast-action dried yeast ....
1 tsp sugar (optional) ....
1 tbsp black treacle ....
1½ tsp sea salt ....
115g/4oz/¾ cup mixed seeds, such as linseed, sesame, pumpkin, hemp, sunflower, chia, poppy ....
1 egg, lightly beaten ....
1 tbsp spelt porridge flakes, for sprinkling....................................

COOKS' TIP
The gluten in spelt flour has different qualities than in wheat so spelt requires less kneading time.

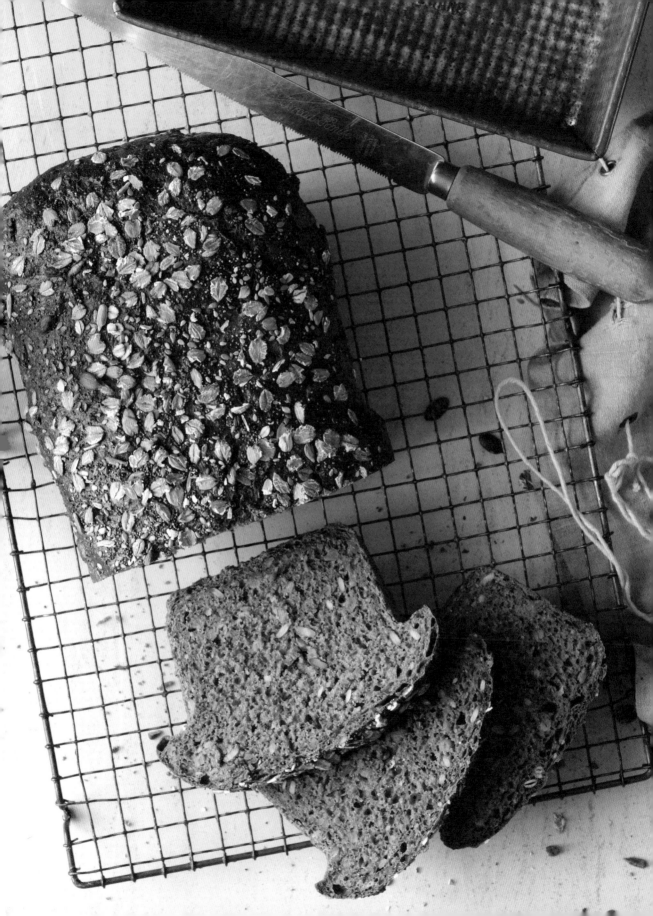

All good artisan bakers have their favourite way of baking a sourdough. The recipe I have chosen below was created by Tom Hitchmough from At the Chapel in Bruton, who bakes the bread for our shop and restaurant at Kilver Court in Somerset.

SOURDOUGH BREAD

MAKES 600g/1lb 5oz loaf
PREPARATION TIME: 20 minutes, plus 2 hours rising and making the starter COOKING TIME: 25 minutes

Lightly oil a baking sheet.

Mix the flour, salt and sourdough starter with 600ml/21fl oz/scant 2½ cups lukewarm water in a large bowl and knead for 10 minutes to a soft dough. Cover with a clean, damp tea towel and leave to rest for 30 minutes. Fold in each corner to the middle and turn the dough upside down, then cover and rest again for 30 minutes. Repeat the folding, turning and resting.

Mould the dough into a loaf, put on the prepared baking sheet, cover and prove for 30–40 minutes. Preheat the oven to 220°C/425°F/Gas 7. Bake for 20–25 minutes until the crust is golden brown and the bread is hollow-sounding when tapped. Transfer to a wire rack to cool.

a little oil, for greasing ....
500g/1lb 2oz/4 cups wholegrain spelt
 flour, plus extra for dusting ....
2 tsp sea salt ....
250g/9oz/1 cup Sourdough Starter
 (see page 17) ....

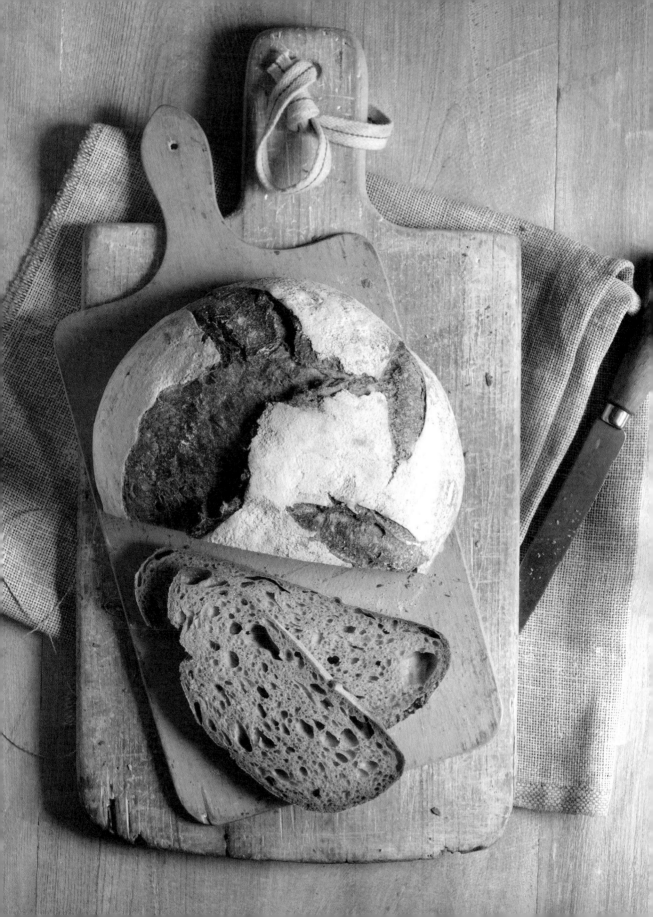

When I first started making bread for the food store Waitrose in London, I found a great baker who would only make my spelt bread for me if he could use a 50/50 rye mix. We did, and it was amazing! Rye lends a pleasing wholesomeness to this easy bread. It is a popular grain across Russia, the Nordic region and Central Europe, and we reckon this dark and rustic bread is a happy marriage of two great grains.

SPELT & RYE BREAD

MAKES 450g/1lb loaf
PREPARATION TIME: 25 minutes, plus 1¾ hours rising COOKING TIME: 1 hour

Lightly oil a large bowl and a baking sheet.

Put all the dry ingredients in another large bowl and make a well in the centre. Add the buttermilk and honey and mix together, using a wooden spoon, to a rough dough.

Turn the dough out onto a lightly floured work surface and knead for 10–12 minutes until the dough is smooth and elastic and springs back when poked. Transfer the kneaded dough to the prepared bowl, cover with a clean, damp tea towel and leave to rise in a warm place for 1 hour, or until doubled in size.

Turn the dough out onto a lightly floured work surface, knock the air out of the dough by punching it with your fist and knead it gently once or twice. Shape the dough into a round ball and put on the prepared baking sheet. Cover again and leave in a warm place for 45 minutes, or until the dough has doubled in size and no longer springs back when poked.

Meanwhile, preheat the oven to 220°C/425°F/Gas 7.

Using a sharp knife, slice three or four diagonal cuts into the top of the dough and brush with either some milk or beaten egg diluted with a little water before sprinkling with some flour and a few spelt and rye flakes, if you like.

Splash a little water in the hot oven to create steam to help the bread to rise. Bake for 15 minutes, then turn the oven down to 190°C/375°F/Gas 5 and bake for a further 30–45 minutes until the bread is just firm and hollow-sounding when tapped. Transfer to a wire rack to cool.

a little oil, for greasing ....
250g/9oz/2 cups white spelt flour ....
125g/4½oz/1 cup wholegrain spelt flour, plus extra for dusting and sprinkling ....
125g/4½oz/1¼ cups rye flour ....
2 tsp sea salt ....
15g/½oz/2 tbsp fresh yeast, crumbled, or 7g/¼oz/2 tsp fast-action dried yeast ....
350ml/12fl oz/1½ cups buttermilk .....
1 tbsp clear honey or black treacle ......
a little milk or beaten egg ....
spelt and rye flakes, for sprinkling (optional) ....

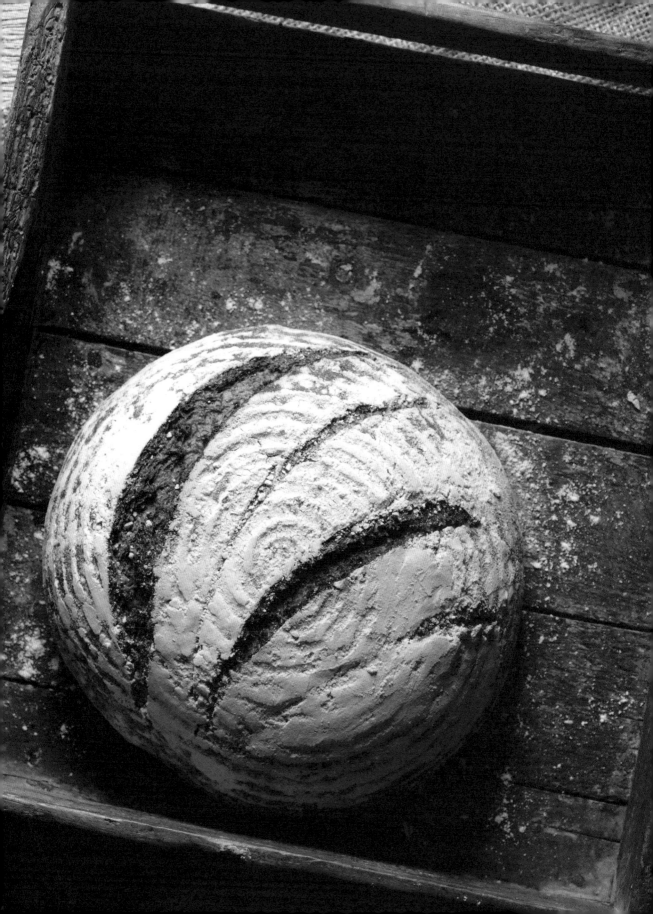

With a wonderful name like ciabatta, you would have thought this rustic bread was born in Tuscany in medieval times. In reality? An Italian baker from near Venice created ciabatta in the 1980s to rival the French baguette, which was over-running Italy as the sandwich bread of choice. What a good job he did, as this light, airy loaf makes the perfect base for your preferred fillings. Our recipe has been created by our favourite Somerset baker, Tom Hitchmough.

CIABATTA

MAKES 500g/1lb 2oz loaf
PREPARATION TIME: 20 minutes, plus 55 minutes resting COOKING TIME: 20 minutes

Lightly grease a 20cm/8in square baking tin.

Put the flour, salt and yeast in a large bowl. Add 325ml/11fl oz/scant 1⅓ cups lukewarm water and the olive oil and mix together, using a wooden spoon, to form a rough dough.

Turn the dough out onto a lightly floured work surface and knead for 5–8 minutes until the dough is smooth and elastic and springs back when poked. It should come away from the surface easily. Roll and shape the dough to fit into the prepared tin.

Cover the dough with a clean, damp tea towel and leave to rise in a warm place for 20 minutes. Fold the left side of the dough into the middle and then repeat with the right side, making sure you trap plenty of air bubbles inside the dough. Carefully turn the dough over and then cover again and leave to stand for a further 20 minutes. Repeat this process three more times, then leave it to rest for a final 10 minutes.

Turn the dough out onto a lightly floured work surface and leave to rest for 2 minutes. Meanwhile, preheat the oven to 250°C/500°F/Gas 9 and put a large baking sheet in the oven to heat up. Turn the dough over so that both sides are floury, then stretch the dough out to a rectangle shape and gently slide it onto the hot baking sheet.

Spray a little water in the hot oven to help the bread to rise and to give the ciabatta a really good crust, then place the bread in the oven and turn the oven down to 220°C/425°F/Gas 7. Bake for 18–20 minutes, or until golden on top and hollow-sounding when tapped. Transfer to a wire rack to cool.

4 tsp olive oil, plus extra for
   greasing ....
500g/1lb 2oz/4 cups white spelt flour,
   plus extra for dusting ....
2 tsp salt...
10g/⅓oz/1 tbsp fresh yeast, crumbled,
   or 7g/¼oz/1 tsp fast-action dried
   yeast ....

English muffins are so simple to prepare and don't require an oven. They're a cross between a dough and a pancake batter, and once you've made this version – with both white and a little wholegrain spelt flour for an extra-wholesome flavour – you'll never be content with shop-bought English muffins again.

ENGLISH MUFFINS

MAKES 10 muffins
PREPARATION TIME: 20 minutes, plus 1½ hours rising   COOKING TIME: 30 minutes per batch

Melt the butter with the milk in a small pan over a low heat, then leave to cool to around 35°C/95°F. Lightly oil a large bowl.

Put all the dry ingredients in another large bowl and make a well in the centre. Add the milk and butter mixture and mix, using a wooden spoon, to form a soft dough.

Turn the dough out onto a lightly floured work surface and knead for 10 minutes, or for 5–7 minutes in a stand mixer with the dough hook attached, until the dough is smooth and elastic and springs back when poked. Transfer the kneaded dough to the prepared bowl, cover with a clean, damp tea towel and leave to rise in a warm place for 1 hour, or until doubled in size.

Turn the dough out again onto a lightly floured work surface, knock the air out of the dough by punching it with your fist and knead gently once or twice, making sure not to punch all the air bubbles out of it, just reshaping it at this stage. Return it to the bowl, cover again and leave to rise in a warm place for a further 20 minutes, or until the dough has doubled in size and no longer springs back when poked.

Carefully divide the dough into 10 evenly sized pieces and gently shape them into balls. Sprinkle some polenta on the work surface and roll the dough in the polenta until each ball is covered and is 1cm/½ inch thick.

Heat a pancake pan or a griddle until it is hot but not smoking. Cook the muffins, a few at a time, for 15 minutes on each side. They should look golden brown and puff up slightly during cooking. Transfer to a wire rack to cool while you cook the remaining muffins. Serve with plenty of good-quality butter.

55g/2oz unsalted butter, plus extra to serve ....
300ml/10½fl oz/1¼cups full-fat milk ....
a little oil, for greasing ....
300g/10½oz/2½ cups white spelt flour ....
150g/5½oz/scant 1¼ cups wholegrain spelt flour ....
1 tsp sea salt ....
¾ tsp golden caster sugar...................
15g/½oz/2 tbsp fresh yeast, crumbled, or 7g/¼oz/2 tsp fast-action dried yeast ....
polenta or semolina, for dusting ....

This is a family favourite. Freddie, my son, has a natural flair for throwing together recipes, and one day this focaccia appeared on the kitchen table – we soon made it disappear! With rosemary and sea salt, this makes a wonderful accompaniment to a meal, or a great starter, dipped in olive oil and balsamic vinegar.

FOCACCIA

MAKES 20 x 30cm/8 x 12in focaccia
PREPARATION TIME: 20 minutes, plus 1¾ hours rising COOKING TIME: 30 minutes

Lightly grease a large mixing bowl. Line a 20 x 30cm/8 x 12in deep-sided baking tin with baking paper and lightly grease this to stop the dough from sticking once baked.

Put the flour, salt and yeast in another large bowl and make a well in the centre. Add the olive oil and 350ml/12fl oz/scant 1½ cups lukewarm water. Mix together, using a wooden spoon or a plastic dough scraper, to a sticky dough.

Turn the dough out onto a greased work surface and knead for about 10 minutes, or until the dough is smooth and elastic and springs back when poked. Transfer the focaccia dough to the prepared bowl, cover with a clean, damp tea towel and leave to rise in a warm place for 1 hour, or until the dough has doubled in size.

Shape the dough in the prepared baking tin, using your hands to spread it into each corner of the tin and prodding it along as you go so that you have little indentations to pour the olive oil into. Take the rosemary sprigs and tear off little bundles, brush these with olive oil to prevent them from burning in the oven and press them into the indentations of the dough. Cover the dough again and leave in a warm place for 30–45 minutes until the dough no longer springs back when poked.

Preheat the oven to 220°C/425°F/Gas 7.

Brush the top of the dough with olive oil, then spread the rest of the oil into the indentations with the rosemary to create little puddles of oil. Sprinkle with sea salt, then bake for 10 minutes. Turn the oven down to 190°C/375°F/Gas 5 and bake for a further 20 minutes, or until the focaccia is golden on top and hollow-sounding when tapped. Leave to cool in the tin for 5 minutes, then transfer to a wire rack to finish cooling.

3 tbsp olive oil, plus extra for greasing ....
500g/1lb 2oz/4 cups white spelt flour ....
2 tsp sea salt, plus extra for sprinkling.................................
30g/1oz/4 tbsp fresh yeast, crumbled, or 14g/½oz/4 tsp fast-action dried yeast ....

FOR THE ROSEMARY GARNISH:
1 bunch of rosemary...........................
3 tbsp olive oil....................................
sea salt ....

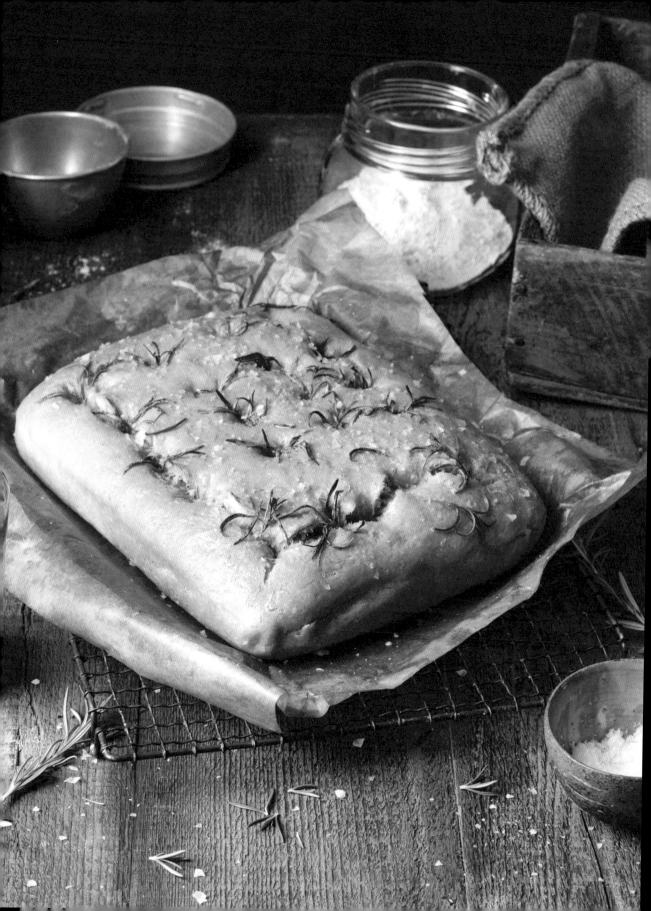

This is a real favourite of mine – a proper Irish soda bread recipe that one of our best friends, Mary Thomas, taught us in the early days of our spelt journey. Mary was doing all the early photography of the produce we were making and the animals we kept at Sharpham Park, and one day just knocked up one of these rustic loaves. If you like a softer crust, try following the Irish tradition of wringing out a wet tea towel until just damp, then wrapping it round the hot soda bread while it cools.

MARY THOMAS' PINE NUT & CRANBERRY SODA BREAD

MAKES 2 x 450g/1lb loaves
PREPARATION TIME: 20 minutes COOKING TIME: 35 minutes

Preheat the oven to 200°C/400°F/Gas 6 and grease a large baking sheet.

Put all the dry ingredients in a large bowl and make a well in the centre. Add the buttermilk, then stir gently with a knife to bind the mixture together to a soft, scone-like consistency, stirring in a little more buttermilk, if needed.

Turn the dough out onto a lightly floured work surface, divide in half and gently shape into rounds. Do not knead or the finished bread will be tough. Slice or press a cross in the top of each loaf, then put on the prepared baking sheet.

Bake for 35 minutes, or until a skewer inserted in the centre comes out clean. Transfer to a wire rack to cool.

a little oil, for greasing ....
675g/1½lb/heaped 5⅓ cups white
  spelt flour, plus extra for dusting......
½ tsp sea salt ....
1 tsp bicarbonate of soda ....
1 handful of pine nuts ....
1 handful of dried cranberries, or any
  dried fruit/seeds of your choice........
285ml/10fl oz/scant 1¼ cups
  buttermilk, plus extra if needed ....

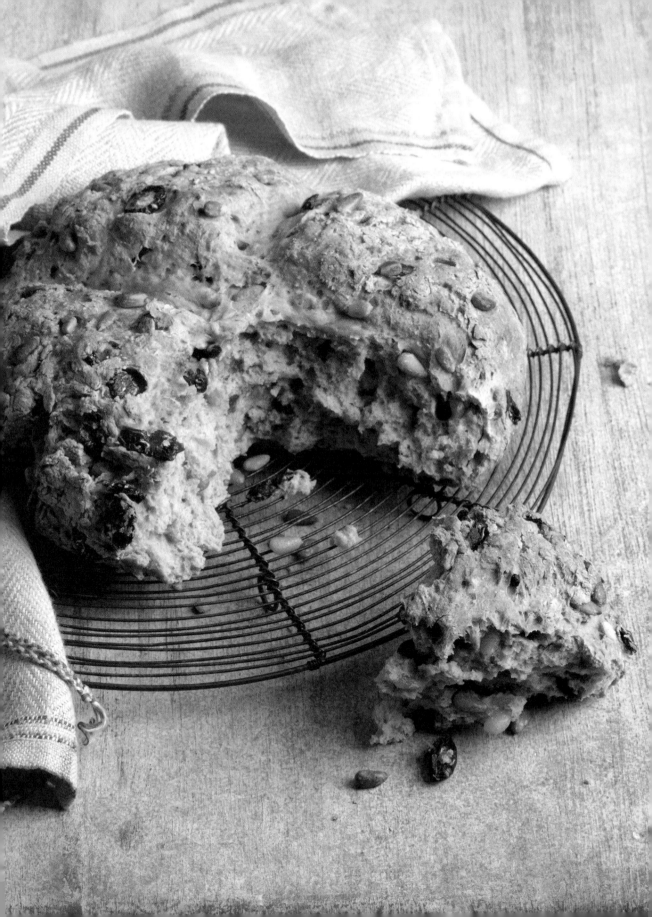

Sweet and savoury at the same time, with an incredible depth of flavour, this quick bread will certainly become a favourite with many of you. The slightly salty tang of the Stilton gives it real depth and perfectly balances the crunch of the walnuts.

WALNUT & STILTON BREAD

MAKES: 900g/2lb loaf
PREPARATION TIME: 30 minutes   COOKING TIME: 40 minutes

Preheat the oven to 200°C/400°F/Gas 6 and lightly oil a baking sheet.

Put half the walnuts into a food processor and whiz until finely ground or crush using a mortar and pestle. Using your hands, break the other pile of walnuts into large, rough chunks.

Put the honey in a small heatproof bowl set over a saucepan of gently simmering water to help loosen it. Add the buttermilk.

Put the flour, bicarbonate of soda, salt and all the walnuts in a large bowl, stir to combine, then make a well in the centre. Add the honey and buttermilk mixture and mix together, using a wooden spoon, to a soft dough. Add the cubes of Stilton and stir to combine again. Don't overmix or the bread will be tough.

Turn the dough out onto a lightly floured work surface, shape it into a round loaf and put on the prepared baking sheet. Slice a deep cross into the top of the bread, cutting almost right the way through to the baking sheet.

Bake for 30–40 minutes until well risen and golden brown. Transfer to a wire rack to cool.

a little oil, for greasing ....
200g/7oz/1⅔ cups walnuts ....
100g/3½oz/⅓ cup clear honey ....
200ml/7fl oz/scant 1 cup
   buttermilk ....
500g/1lb 2oz/4 cups wholegrain
   spelt flour ....
1 tsp bicarbonate of soda ....
1½ tsp salt...
150g/5½oz Stilton cheese, diced.........

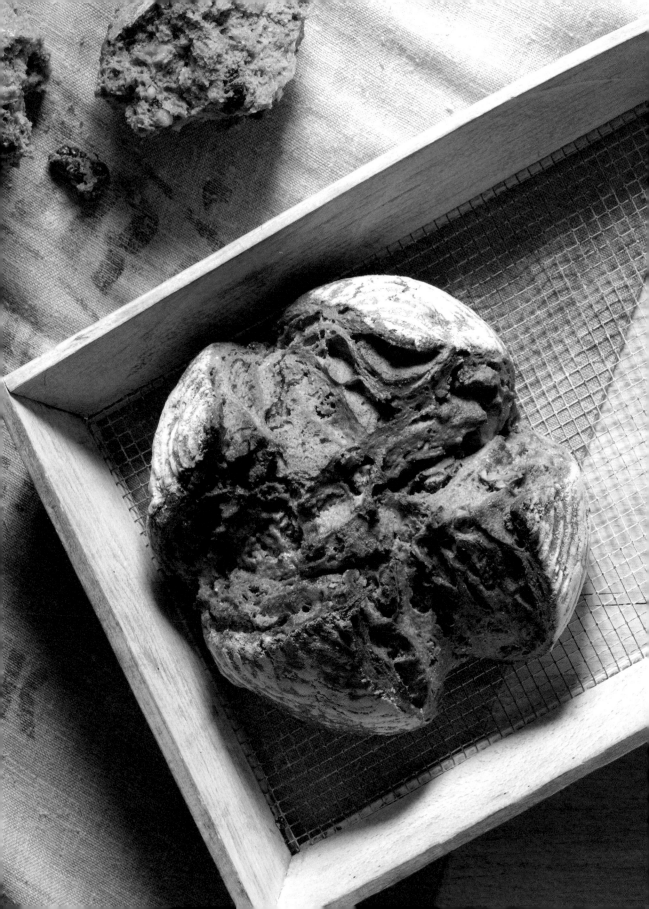

Malt lends a special flavour and sticky quality to this sweet bread. We've gone for a classic combination of raisins and currants but you can, of course, use whatever dried fruit you have to hand. Dates, cranberries, sour cherries, apricots, pears, apples and prunes would all be delicious in this bread. Soaking the raisins and currants in hot water for 10 minutes before adding them to the dough makes the fruit extra plump. You could also soak them in a tea of your choice, and use a mixture of wholegrain and white spelt flour instead of just refined flour, if you like.

FRUIT & MALT BREAD

MAKES 900g/2lb loaf
PREPARATION TIME: 20 minutes, plus 1½ hours rising COOKING TIME: 45 minutes

Lightly oil a large bowl.

Put the flour, yeast, malt extract and salt in another large bowl and make a well in the centre. Pour in 200ml/7fl oz/scant 1 cup lukewarm water and mix together, using a wooden spoon, to a rough dough.

Turn the dough out onto a lightly floured work surface and knead for about 8 minutes, or until the dough is smooth and elastic and springs back when poked. Transfer the kneaded dough to the prepared bowl, cover with a clean, damp tea towel and leave to rise in a warm place for 45 minutes, or until doubled in size.

Meanwhile, preheat the oven to 200°C/400°F/Gas 6 and lightly oil a 900g/2lb loaf tin. Soak the raisins and currants in hot water for 10 minutes, then drain well.

Turn the dough out onto a lightly floured work surface, sprinkle with the dried fruit and knead the dough very gently to incorporate the fruit evenly through the dough. It will be quite messy but persist for a couple of minutes. Mould the dough into a log shape, then put in the prepared loaf tin. Cover again, then leave in a warm place for a further 30–45 minutes until the dough has doubled in size and no longer springs back when poked.

Bake for 45 minutes, or until the bread is golden brown and hollow-sounding when tapped. Turn out onto a wire rack to cool.

While the bread is cooling, put the sugar in a small bowl, pour over 3 tablespoons hot water and stir until dissolved. Brush this over the loaf while it is still warm. Serve the loaf sliced and buttered.

a little oil, for greasing......................
500g/1lb 2oz/4 cups white spelt flour,
    plus extra for dusting......................
15g/½oz/2 tbsp fresh yeast,
    crumbled, or 7g/¼oz/2 tsp fast-
    action dried yeast..........................
3 tbsp malt extract............................
1 tsp sea salt ....
90g/3¼oz/¾ cup raisins ....
90g/3¼oz/¾ cup currants ....
1 tbsp light soft brown sugar ....
unsalted butter, to serve.....................

COOKS' TIP
This bread stores exceptionally well. Keep it well wrapped in the fridge and it will last for about three weeks – if you can resist it for that long, of course.

Stollen is a traditional Christmas bread from Germany. In Dresden, in 1730, a giant 1.7-ton stollen was ordered by the king to feed 24,000 guests at a feast! This fruit and nut sourdough bread recipe is a modification of the traditional bread. It uses the principle that the fermentation process both predigests the proteins and starches, and neutralizes anti-nutrients, compounds that interfere with the efficient absorption of nutrients. This makes the nutrients in the foods easier to digest and therefore makes the stollen more digestible and nutritious. It's well worth the effort for both the complex flavour generated by the starter and also for the health benefits.

SOURDOUGH STOLLEN

MAKES 30 x 13cm/12 x 5in loaf
PREPARATION TIME: 1 hour, plus 24 hours soaking and 16 hours proving COOKING TIME: **30 minutes**

In a large bowl, mix together the spices, orange and lemon zest, orange juice, kefir, cherries, almonds, raisins, rum and port. Cover with a tea towel and leave to soak for 12–24 hours.

Grease and flour a large baking sheet.

Put the flour and salt in a large bowl, then rub in the butter, using your fingertips, until the mixture resembles fine breadcrumbs. Stir in the honey, then the egg. Add the marinated fruit and nuts and sourdough starter and mix together, using a wooden spoon, to a rough dough.

Turn the dough out onto a lightly floured work surface and knead until the dough is smooth and pliable, adding a little milk or flour, if necessary. The fruit and nuts make it a little challenging to knead but persevere for 5 minutes, or until the dough has a satin-like finish.

Shape the dough into a log and pat down into a flat, oval shape about 25 x 8cm/10 x 3¼in and 5cm/2in thick. Put the dough in the centre of the prepared baking sheet. As the dough rises, it will tend to spread so the final stollen will be much wider. Cover with a clean, damp tea towel and leave in a warm place (ideally at 28–32°C/82–90°F) for 12–16 hours until it has doubled in size. If the weather is hot you may need to remoisten the tea towel periodically. If the surface dries out and forms a dry crust, then it will prevent the dough from rising.

Preheat the oven to 180°C/350°F/Gas 4.

Bake the loaf for 25–30 minutes, or until a knife inserted in the centre comes out clean. Brush with the melted butter as soon as you remove it from the oven. Transfer to a wire rack to cool.

½ tsp mixed spice ....
¼ tsp ground cinnamon ....
⅛ tsp freshly grated nutmeg ....
⅛ tsp ground cardamom ....
grated zest of 1 small orange ....
1 tbsp grated lemon zest ....
4 tbsp orange juice ....
2 tbsp kefir or a plain probiotic milk
    or yogurt drink ....
60g/2¼oz/¼ cup cherries (fresh if
    possible), pitted ....
60g/2¼oz/½ cup almonds, flaked or
    chopped..
125g/4½oz/1 cup raisins ....
1 tbsp dark rum...............................
1 tbsp port or sherry.........................
150g/5½oz unsalted butter, softened,
    plus extra for greasing and 2 tbsp,
    melted and cooled, for brushing ......
600g/1lb 5oz/4¾ cups white spelt
    flour, plus extra for dusting.............
¼ tsp sea salt ....
60g/2¼oz/2½ tbsp clear honey ....
1 egg, beaten ....
60g/2¼oz/¼ cup Sourdough Starter
    (see page 17).................................
a little milk, if needed........................

A kringle is a circular or knot-shaped Scandinavian pastry. This show-stopper recipe, inspired by the great tradition of Baltic baking, comes to us from Brendan Lynch, a contestant on the BBC television show *The Great British Bake Off*, and is flavoured with the perfect pairing of orange and cinnamon.

BALTIC ORANGE & CINNAMON KRINGLE BREAD

MAKES 23cm/9in loaf
PREPARATION TIME: 25 minutes, plus 1½ hours rising   COOKING TIME: 35 minutes

Lightly grease a large bowl and a baking sheet. Put the flours, salt, yeast, orange zest and sugar in another large bowl and make a well in the centre. Mix together the remaining kringle ingredients in a smaller bowl. Pour the liquid ingredients into the dry ingredients and mix together, using a wooden spoon, to a rough dough.

Turn the dough out onto a lightly floured work surface and knead for about 5 minutes, or until the dough is smooth and elastic and springs back when poked. Transfer the kneaded dough to the prepared bowl, cover with a clean, damp tea towel and leave to rise in a warm place for 1 hour, or until doubled in size.

Turn the dough out onto a lightly floured work surface and roll out to a 50 x 36cm/20 x 14in rectangle 1cm/½in thick. For the cinnamon filling, spread most of the melted butter across the dough. Mix the sugar and cinnamon, reserve 1 tablespoon, then sprinkle the rest over the dough. Roll up the dough from the long side into a fairly tight log, then cut in half lengthways. Keep the exposed cuts on the top and twist the two halves together firmly into a circle about 23cm/9in in diameter, sealing the ends together with a little water. Put the dough on the prepared baking sheet, brush with the remaining melted butter and sprinkle with the reserved cinnamon sugar. Leave uncovered in a warm place for 30 minutes. Preheat the oven to 220°C/425°F/Gas 7.

Bake for 5 minutes, then turn the oven down to 180°C/350°F/Gas 4 and bake for a further 25–30 minutes until golden brown. Transfer to a wire rack to cool.

For the icing, put the icing sugar in a small bowl and gradually add enough orange juice to mix to a fairly thick consistency. Stir in the orange zest, if using, for extra flavour. Drizzle the icing over the kringle.

FOR THE ORANGE KRINGLE:
30g/1oz unsalted butter, melted and cooled, plus extra for greasing ....
175g/6oz/1⅓ cups white spelt flour, plus extra for dusting ....
130g/4½oz/heaped 1 cup wholegrain spelt flour ....
½ tsp salt ....
15g/½oz/2 tbsp fresh yeast, crumbled, or 7g/¼oz/2 tsp fast-action dried yeast ....
finely grated zest of 1 large orange
1 tbsp caster sugar ....
160ml/5¼fl oz/⅔ cup lukewarm full-fat milk..
1 egg yolk...
½ tsp orange flower water (optional) ..

FOR THE CINNAMON FILLING:
60g/2¼oz unsalted butter, melted and cooled..
4 tbsp golden caster sugar ....
1 tbsp ground cinnamon ....

FOR THE ORANGE ICING:
30g/1oz/¼ cup icing sugar, sifted ....
a few squeezes of fresh orange juice.....
1 tbsp very finely chopped orange zest (optional) ....

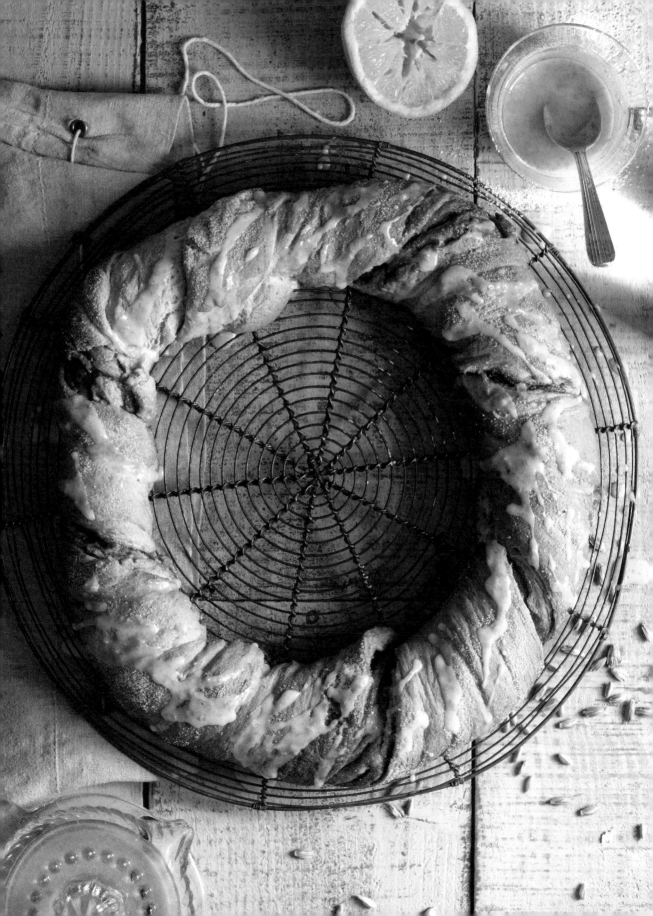

These little buns are great for those avoiding refined sugars. The honey lends just enough sweetness, while the tartness of the sour cherries balances the warm, spicy flavours, making them perfect for elevenses. For a change, try using other dried fruits, or sprinkling some desiccated coconut on the top. Nuts or citrus zest make great additions, too.

HONEY & SOUR CHERRY BUNS

MAKES 8 buns
PREPARATION TIME: 30 minutes, plus 1 hour rising   COOKING TIME: 25 minutes

Lightly grease a large bowl and line a baking sheet with baking paper.

Sift all the dry ingredients together into another large bowl and make a well in the centre. Add the buttermilk, butter, 1 egg and half the honey and mix together, using a wooden spoon, to a rough dough.

Turn the dough out onto a lightly floured work surface and knead for 8 minutes, or until the dough is smooth and elastic and springs back when poked. Transfer the kneaded dough to the prepared bowl, cover with a clean, damp tea towel and leave to rise in a warm place for 30 minutes, or until doubled in size. Meanwhile, put the cherries in a bowl, cover with hot water and leave to soak.

Turn the dough out onto a lightly floured work surface and gently knock the air out of the dough by punching it with your fist, but make sure not to squash all the air bubbles out of it.

Drain the cherries of their soaking liquid and scatter them over the dough. Carefully bring the dough together and knead the fruit gently into the dough. Shape and roll into 8 buns, then put on the prepared baking sheet. Cover with a clean, damp tea towel and leave to rise in a warm place for a further 20–30 minutes until the dough has doubled in size again and no longer springs back when poked.

Preheat the oven to 220°C/425°F/Gas 7.

Beat the remaining egg and brush it over the risen buns. Spray a little water in the hot oven to create steam to help the buns to rise. Bake on the middle shelf for 5 minutes, then turn the oven down to 180°C/350°F/Gas 4 and bake for a further 15–20 minutes until the buns are golden and hollow-sounding when tapped. Transfer to a wire rack to cool. While still warm, brush with the remaining honey to glaze. If the honey is thick, dilute with 1–2 teaspoons boiling water.

a little oil, for greasing ....
350g/12oz/2¾ cups white spelt flour, plus extra for dusting ....
115g/4oz/scant 1 cup wholegrain spelt flour ....
1½ tsp mixed spice ....
1 tsp sea salt ....
15g/½oz/2 tbsp fresh yeast, crumbled, or 7g/¼oz/2 tsp fast-action dried yeast ....
250ml/9fl oz/1 cup buttermilk, at room temperature ....
55g/2oz unsalted butter, melted and cooled ....
2 eggs, lightly beaten ....
4 tbsp clear honey ....
150g/5½oz/scant 1¼ cups dried sour cherries ....

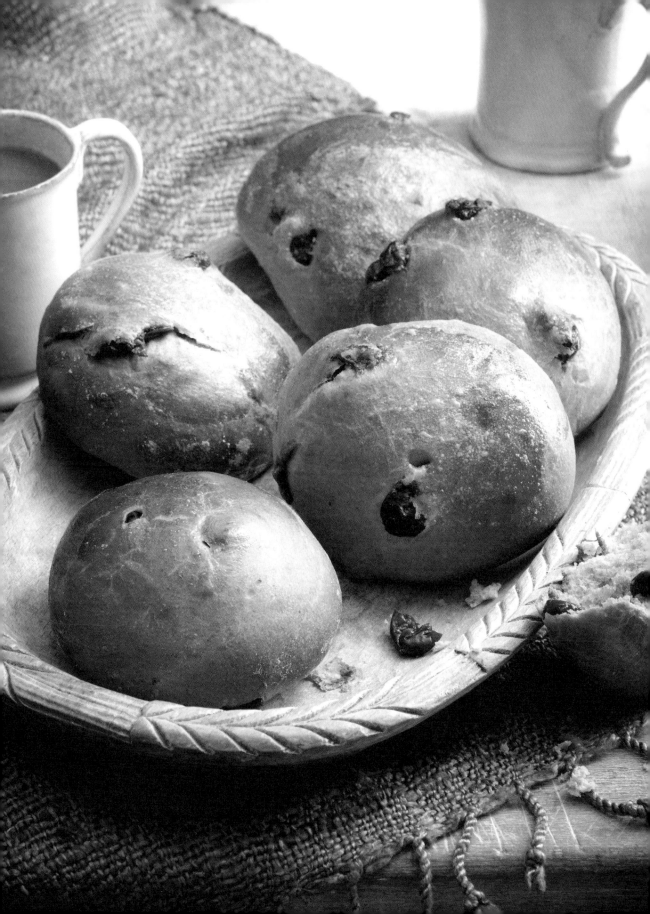

Enriched buns made with yeast are commonplace in Scandinavia, and spelt flour makes these buns soft and utterly moreish. They're not too sweet but have lots of flavour from the cardamom and the almonds. Using freshly ground cardamom seeds from green cardamom pods is best – the ground spices in supermarkets don't have as much flavour.

SCANDINAVIAN CARDAMOM & ALMOND TWISTS

MAKES 8–10 twists
PREPARATION TIME: 30 minutes, plus 50 minutes rising COOKING TIME: 25 minutes

Lightly grease a large bowl and line a baking sheet with baking paper.

Put the flours, sugar, cardamom, salt and yeast in another large bowl and make a well in the centre. Add the milk, butter and egg and mix together, using a wooden spoon, to a soft dough.

Turn the dough out onto a lightly floured work surface and knead for about 8 minutes, or until the dough is soft and elastic and springs back when poked. Transfer the kneaded dough to the prepared bowl, cover with a clean, damp tea towel and leave to rise in a warm place for 30 minutes, or until it has doubled in size.

Turn the dough out onto a lightly floured work surface and roll out to a 35 x 25cm/14 x 10in rectangle. Spread the butter for the filling evenly over half the dough in a long strip, then scatter the remaining filling ingredients on top. Fold over the unfilled half of the dough across the filling, closing it like a book. Using a sharp, non-serrated knife, cut the dough into 8–10 even slices. Hold each end of a slice and twist it 3 or 4 times, then knot the dough and put on the prepared baking sheet. Repeat with the remaining twists, spacing them a little way apart. Cover as before and leave to rise in a warm place for 20 minutes, or until they have doubled in size and no longer spring back when poked.

Preheat the oven to 220°C/425°F/Gas 7.

Brush the risen buns with the beaten egg and scatter the flaked almonds on top. Spray a little water in the hot oven to create steam to help the buns to rise. Bake on the middle shelf for 5 minutes, then turn the oven down to 180°C/350°F/Gas 4 and bake for a further 15–20 minutes until the buns are golden and hollow-sounding when tapped. Transfer to a wire rack to cool.

55g/2oz unsalted butter, melted and cooled, plus extra for greasing..........
350g/12oz/2¾ cups white spelt flour, plus extra for dusting ....
115g/4oz/scant 1 cup wholegrain spelt flour ....
55g/2oz/¼ cup caster sugar ....
1½ tsp freshly ground cardamom ....
1 tsp sea salt ....
15g/½oz/2 tbsp fresh yeast, crumbled, or 7g/¼oz/2 tsp fast-action dried yeast ....
250ml/9fl oz/1 cup full-fat milk, lukewarm...
1 egg, beaten ....

FOR THE CARDAMOM & ALMOND FILLING:
75g/2½oz unsalted butter, softened....
55g/2oz/scant ⅓ cup light brown muscovado sugar............................
55g/2oz /⅓ cup whole almonds, skin on, crushed or ground ....
2 tsp freshly ground cardamom ....
1 tsp vanilla extract............................

FOR THE TOPPING:
1 egg, beaten ....
55g/2oz/½ cup flaked almonds..........

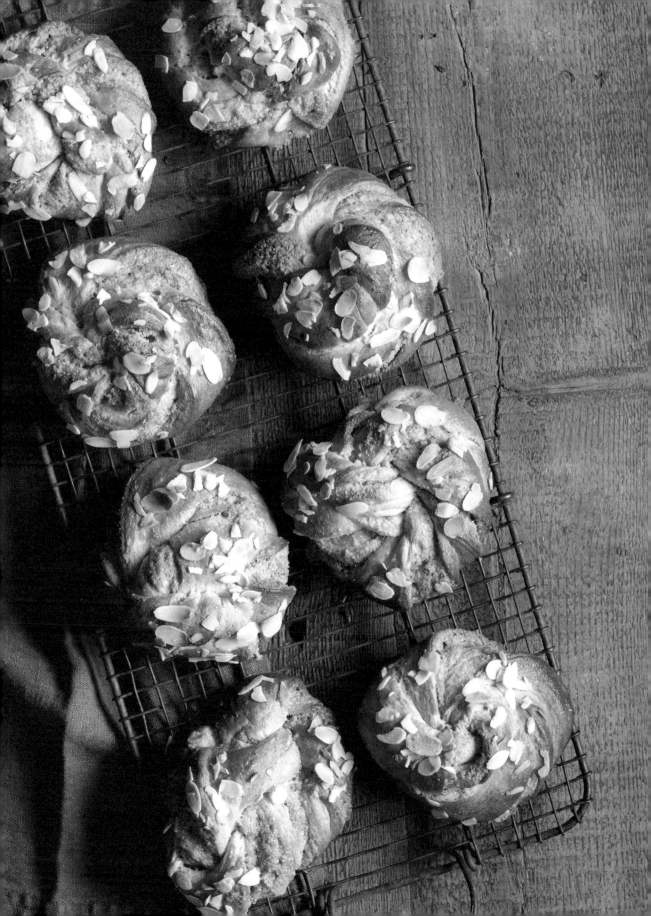

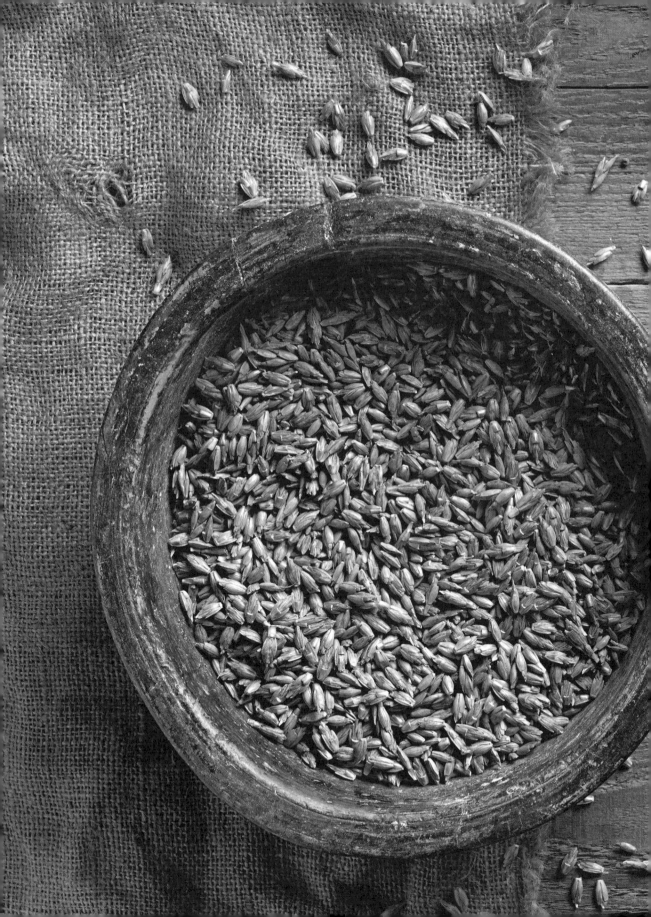

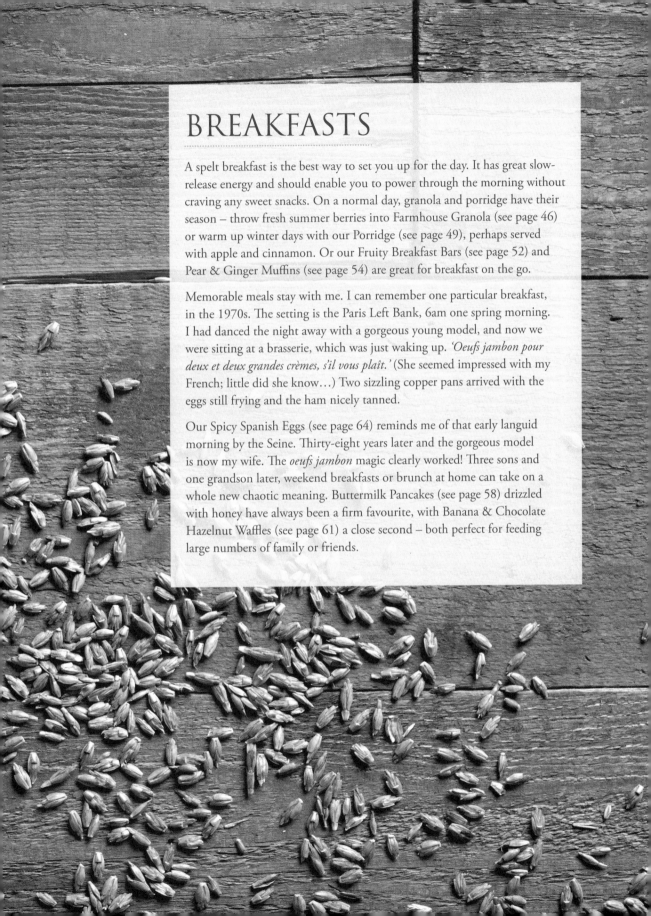

BREAKFASTS

A spelt breakfast is the best way to set you up for the day. It has great slow-release energy and should enable you to power through the morning without craving any sweet snacks. On a normal day, granola and porridge have their season – throw fresh summer berries into Farmhouse Granola (see page 46) or warm up winter days with our Porridge (see page 49), perhaps served with apple and cinnamon. Or our Fruity Breakfast Bars (see page 52) and Pear & Ginger Muffins (see page 54) are great for breakfast on the go.

Memorable meals stay with me. I can remember one particular breakfast, in the 1970s. The setting is the Paris Left Bank, 6am one spring morning. I had danced the night away with a gorgeous young model, and now we were sitting at a brasserie, which was just waking up. *'Oeufs jambon pour deux et deux grandes crèmes, s'il vous plaît.'* (She seemed impressed with my French; little did she know…) Two sizzling copper pans arrived with the eggs still frying and the ham nicely tanned.

Our Spicy Spanish Eggs (see page 64) reminds me of that early languid morning by the Seine. Thirty-eight years later and the gorgeous model is now my wife. The *oeufs jambon* magic clearly worked! Three sons and one grandson later, weekend breakfasts or brunch at home can take on a whole new chaotic meaning. Buttermilk Pancakes (see page 58) drizzled with honey have always been a firm favourite, with Banana & Chocolate Hazelnut Waffles (see page 61) a close second – both perfect for feeding large numbers of family or friends.

We have spent years perfecting our Sharpham Park granola and my favourite is our Farmhouse variety, which has just the right balance of nuts, honey and spelt. Remember that the type of honey you use can make all the difference, as bees collect their nectar through the year from local sources, so all sorts of different scents and tastes come through in the various varieties. My first choice is acacia-based honey – light, sweet and fragrant.

FARMHOUSE GRANOLA

MAKES about 450g/1lb
PREPARATION TIME: 10 minutes COOKING TIME: 30 minutes

Preheat the oven to 140°C/275°F/Gas 1 and lightly grease a 20 x 30cm/8 x 12in roasting tin with oil or line with baking paper.

Put the spelt porridge flakes, nuts and seeds in a large bowl and mix together well. In a separate bowl, mix together the oil, honey, vanilla and salt, then pour the mixture into the dry ingredients. Stir well to combine the ingredients and coat the flakes and nuts in the honey and oil. Spread the mixture evenly in the roasting tin.

Bake for 10 minutes, then stir the granola to make sure it will cook evenly. Return it to the oven for a further 20 minutes, or until golden and crunchy.

Leave to cool, then transfer the granola to an airtight container. Add the dried fruit to the mixture and shake well to distribute the fruit. Enjoy with Greek yogurt or ice-cold milk in the morning, or as a snack in the afternoon.

2 tbsp sunflower oil, plus extra for greasing (optional) ....
250g/9oz/2½ cups spelt porridge flakes, toasted ....
55g/2oz/heaped ⅓ cup unsalted mixed nuts, such as any combination of almonds, hazelnuts, pecans, walnuts
55g/2oz/scant ½ cup sunflower seeds ....
55g/2oz/scant ½ cup pumpkin seeds ....
55g/2oz/2½ tbsp clear honey ....
2 tsp vanilla extract...........................
a pinch of sea salt ....
55–115g/2–4oz/½–1 cup mixed dried fruit such as raisins, sour cherries, mango, banana, pineapple, coconut flakes ....
Greek yogurt or ice-cold milk, to serve ....

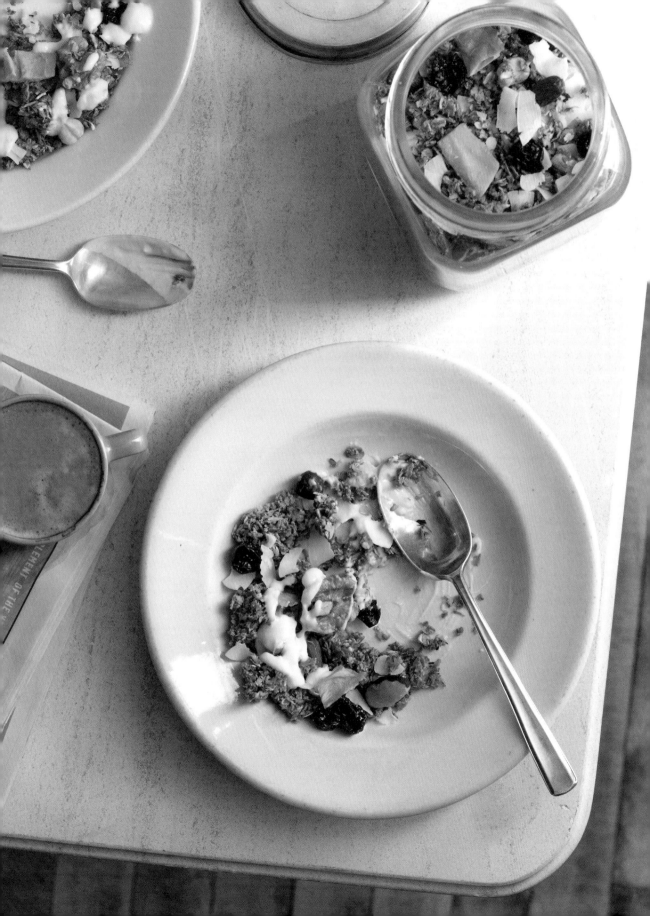

This makes a few weeks' supply of muesli, so make sure it stays fresh by keeping it in an airtight container. The great thing about making your own muesli is you can play around with the ingredients and add whatever you like. This is a wholesome version with no added sugar but natural sweetness from the dried fruit, plus loads of nutrients from the spelt, nuts and seeds. You can vary the flavours, adding spices such as cinnamon and changing the fruit, seed and nut selection depending on what you have in your store cupboard.

MONTY'S MUESLI

MAKES 1.25kg/2lb 12oz
PREPARATION TIME: 10 minutes

Simply mix all the ingredients together in a large, airtight container, pop the lid on and shake the muesli around so that you distribute the ingredients evenly.

Serve with milk of your choice.

500g/1lb 2 oz/5 cups spelt porridge flakes ....
200g/7oz unsalted nuts of your choice, such as almonds, walnuts, cashews, hazelnuts, pecans ....
200g/7oz/1⅔ cups dried fruit, such as sour cherries, raisins, apricots, pitted dates, mango, pineapple, apple ....
100g/3½oz/heaped ¾ cup pumpkin seeds ....
100g/3½oz/⅔ cup linseeds ....
100g/3½oz/1 cup coconut flakes or shavings (optional).........................
spices and flavourings of your choice (optional) ....
milk, to serve.....................................

SWISS-STYLE BIRCHER MUESLI
To make a delicious Swiss-style Bircher muesli, put a portion of this spelt muesli in a bowl, then grate an apple into the bowl, add a spoonful of natural probiotic yogurt and soak with either water, apple juice or milk of your choice. Cover with cling film and keep chilled in the fridge for up to 5 days. This makes a great alternative to wintery porridge and is thought to be an extra-digestible version of muesli.

Spelt porridge, like its oaty cousin, is the breakfast of champions. A fantastic source of slow-release energy and packed full of nutrients, this is a favourite of Arctic explorers. This recipes makes a single portion but it is easy to scale it up depending on how many people you are feeding for breakfast. It tastes excellent with poached apricot and ginger topping (see page 61).

PORRIDGE

MAKES 1 portion
PREPARATION TIME: 5 minutes COOKING TIME: 10 minutes

Put the spelt porridge flakes and milk in a small saucepan over a medium heat and add the salt, if you like. Bring to a gentle simmer and cook for 6 minutes, or until the porridge is creamy, stirring occasionally.

Serve drizzled with the honey, grated apple, seasonal berries and nuts and seeds of your choice.

55g/2oz/heaped ½ cup spelt porridge
    flakes ....
220ml/7½fl oz/scant 1 cup full-fat
    milk or water ....
a pinch of salt (optional) ....

FOR THE TOPPING:
1 tbsp clear honey ....
1 apple, peeled, cored and grated........
1 handful of seasonal berries...............
1 handful of nuts or seeds...................

DAIRY-FREE PORRIDGE

For a dairy-free version of this porridge, try cooking the spelt porridge flakes in coconut milk or cream. You could also add some dried fruit such as raisins, sultanas or chopped dried pear to the porridge just before the end of the cooking time. A scattering of spelt granola on top with some fruit compôte also makes a great textural contrast.

Angela has been a tremendous supporter of our spelt endeavours over the years and really enjoys using spelt products in her cooking. This is her recipe and is just delicious. It is also really quick and easy to make so do give it a try.

ANGELA HARTNETT'S BANANA BREAKFAST LOAF

MAKES 900g/2lb loaf
PREPARATION TIME: 15 minutes COOKING TIME: 45 minutes

Preheat the oven to 180°C/350°F/Gas 4 and line a 900g/2lb loaf tin with baking paper.

Mash the bananas in a large bowl, then add the sugar and eggs and mix until well blended. Add the flours, salt, bicarbonate of soda and ground walnuts and stir until well blended. Stir in the butter, then quickly pour the mixture into the prepared loaf tin and bake for 45 minutes, or until the bread is risen, golden brown and firm to the touch. Transfer to a wire rack to cool.

2–3 ripe bananas ....
150g/5½oz/heaped ⅔ cup golden caster or heaped ¾ cup light brown muscovado sugar...........................
2 eggs, lightly beaten ....
75g/2½oz/heaped ½ cup wholegrain spelt flour ....
55g/2oz/scant ½ cup white spelt flour ....
½ tsp sea salt ....
½ tsp bicarbonate of soda ....
65g/2¼oz/⅔ cup ground walnuts.......
25g/1oz butter, melted and cooled .....

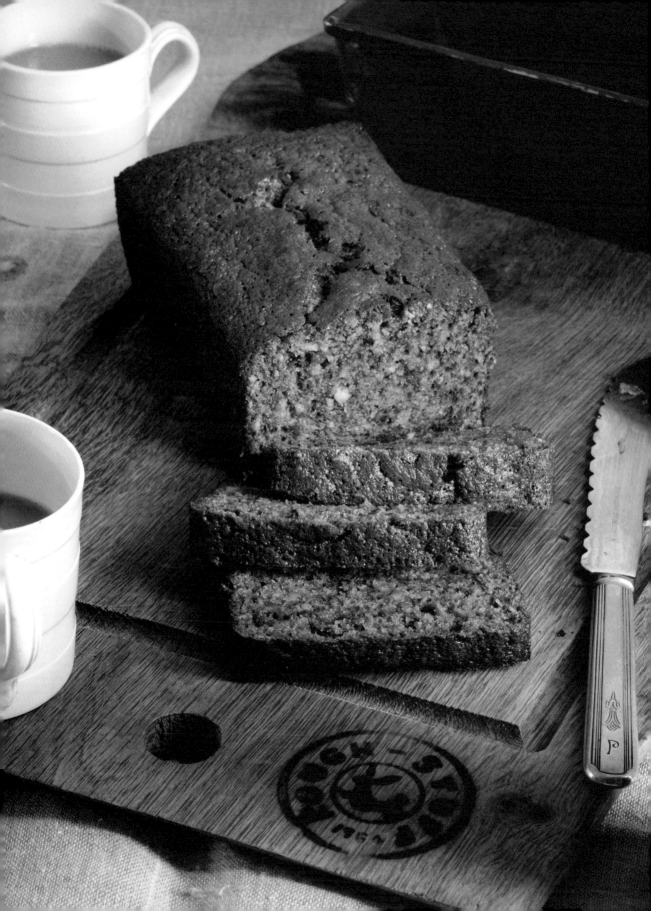

We love these snack bars from Jessica Andersson, a great nutritionist and friend of Sharpham Park who kindly gave us this recipe for the Bowel Cancer Campaign to raise awareness about eating a high-fibre diet. They contain no added refined sugar, the sweetness coming from a little honey and molasses. Bake a batch, stick them in a tin and take one 'to go' for an energy boost on the run.

FRUITY BREAKFAST BARS

MAKES **10 bars**
PREPARATION TIME: **10 minutes** COOKING TIME: **20 minutes**

Preheat the oven to 180°C/350°F/Gas 5. Lightly grease a 15 x 20cm/ 6 x 8in baking tin and line with baking paper, if you like, making sure it hangs a little over the edges, then lightly grease the paper.

Mix together the spelt porridge flakes, flour, seeds, cinnamon and chopped fruit in a large bowl. Melt the butter and molasses in a small saucepan over a low heat. Add the butter mixture to the dry ingredients with the honey and vanilla and mix together well. Spoon the mixture into the prepared tin and, using a potato masher, press it evenly into the tin.

Bake for 20 minutes until the mixture is golden in colour. Leave to cool completely in the tin, then remove and cut into 10 bars. Store in an airtight container.

100g/3½oz unsalted butter, plus extra for greasing.......................................
150g/5½oz/1½ cups spelt porridge flakes ....
2 tbsp wholegrain spelt flour ....
80g/2¾oz/½ cup mixed seeds, such as pumpkin or sesame..............
1 tsp ground cinnamon ....
100g/3½oz/heaped ¾ cup chopped dried fruit, such as pitted and chopped apricots, dates, cranberries ....
1 tbsp molasses..................................
3 tbsp clear honey ....
1 tsp vanilla extract............................

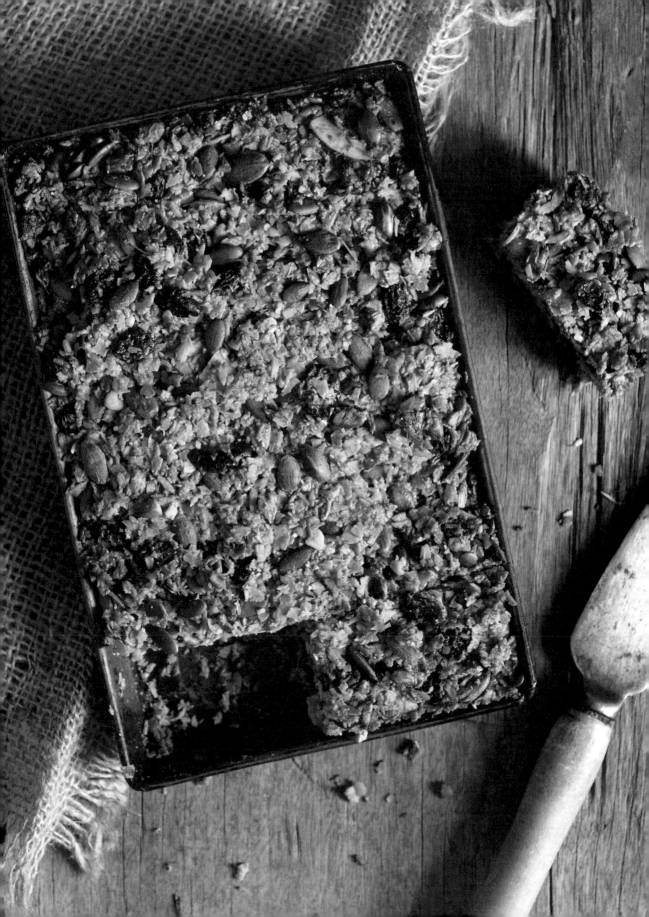

This delicious recipe makes a firm-textured muffin and comes courtesy of Amanda Hamilton, a power-house of a nutritionist and broadcaster who contributed this to the Great British Spelt Recipes campaign. You can use baby fruit purée instead of pear purée, if you like. The muffins make a great on-the-go breakfast with an extra pot of natural yogurt or a piece of fruit, and are especially convenient as you can make them in advance and freeze them. Simply take one out to defrost overnight ready to be reheated in a warm oven or in the microwave in the morning.

PEAR & GINGER MUFFINS

MAKES 12 muffins
PREPARATION TIME: 15 minutes   COOKING TIME: 25 minutes

Preheat the oven to 190°C/375°F/Gas 6 and grease a 12-hole muffin tin or line with squares of baking paper.

Put the flour, oats, baking powder, bicarbonate of soda and spices in a large bowl and make a well in the centre. In a separate bowl, mix together the pear purée, egg whites, yogurt and honey. Pour the liquid ingredients into the well in the dry ingredients and gently fold together to combine, being careful not to overmix. You should have a cake-like batter. Gently fold in the sultanas and diced pear. Do not overmix or your muffins will be tough. Spoon the mixture into the prepared muffin tin.

Bake for 20–25 minutes until well risen and springy to the touch. Transfer to a wire rack to cool for 5 minutes before unwrapping.

a little unsalted butter, for greasing (optional) ....
150g/5½oz/scant 1¼ cups wholegrain or seeded spelt flour ....
150g/5½oz/1½ cups rolled oats..........
2 tsp baking powder ....
1 tsp bicarbonate of soda ....
1 tsp ground ginger ....
1 tsp ground cinnamon ....
¼ tsp freshly grated nutmeg ....
225g/8oz/scant 1 cup pear purée ....
4 egg whites..
125g/4½oz/½ cup natural yogurt.......
200g/7oz/scant 1 cup clear honey.......
115g/4oz/scant 1 cup sultanas............
1 firm pear, peeled, cored and diced ...

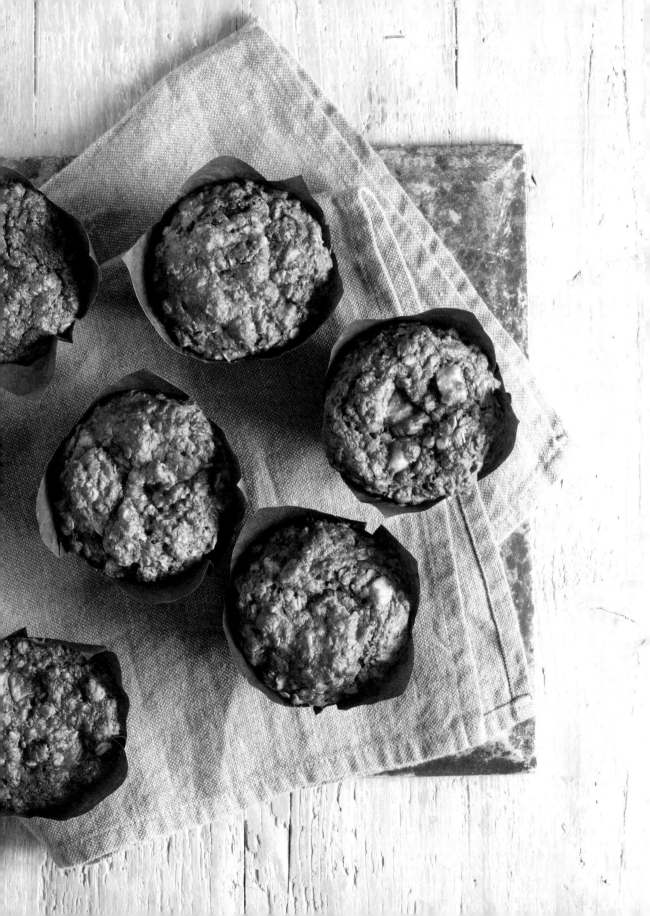

These light and fruity muffins contain chia seeds. The seeds are cultivated on the sierras of South America, where the plants have been grown for thousands of years and once formed an integral part of the Aztec and Mayan diets. Chia seeds are packed full of omega-3, calcium and iron.

BLUEBERRY, LEMON & CHIA SEED MUFFINS

MAKES 6 large muffins
PREPARATION TIME: 15 minutes COOKING TIME: 20 minutes

Preheat the oven to 190°C/375°F/Gas 5 and grease a 6-hole muffin tin or line with paper cases.

Put the flour, baking powder and salt in a large bowl and make a well in the centre. In a separate bowl, combine the buttermilk, melted butter, sugar, lemon zest and juice and egg. Pour the liquid ingredients into the well in the dry ingredients and gently fold together to combine, being careful not to overmix. Gently fold in the blueberries and chia seeds. Quickly spoon the mixture into the prepared muffin cases.

Bake for 20 minutes, or until the muffins are well risen, golden and springy to the touch. Transfer to a wire rack to cool.

100g/3½oz unsalted butter, melted and cooled, plus extra for greasing (optional) ....
160g/5¾oz/1¼ cups white spelt flour
1 tsp baking powder ....
a pinch of salt ....
170ml/5½fl oz/⅔ cup buttermilk ....
60g/2¼oz/heaped ¼ cup caster sugar ....
grated zest and juice of 1 lemon ....
1 egg, lightly beaten ....
140g/5oz/scant 1 cup blueberries ....
55g/2oz/⅓ cup chia seeds.................

Also known as *pain perdu*, this is based on an old recipe that uses stale spelt bread as a base, but really comes alive again with eggs, milk, brown sugar and, of course, fruit and lots more. You can make the berry compôte in advance, if you wish.

VANILLA FRENCH TOAST WITH SUMMER BERRY COMPÔTE

SERVES 4

PREPARATION TIME: **20 minutes** COOKING TIME: **15 minutes**

Preheat the oven to its lowest setting.

Put the eggs, milk, brown sugar, vanilla and salt in a large bowl and whisk until combined. Dunk the bread slices into the egg mixture and allow them to soak up the egg for a few minutes.

Cook the French toast in batches, depending on the size of your pan. Heat a little of the oil and butter in a pancake pan or frying pan over a medium heat until foaming hot. Lift the bread slices out of the egg mixture, allowing any excess liquid to drip back into the bowl before putting them in the pan. Fry for 1–2 minutes on each side until the bread is golden brown. Transfer to a serving plate and keep the French toast warm in the oven while you fry the remaining slices.

Meanwhile, to make the berry topping, put the summer berries in a saucepan over a medium heat with about 150ml/5fl oz/scant ⅔ cup water and heat gently until the berries start to burst and bleed. Turn the heat up to high and let the fruit come to the boil, then add the sugar and stir to combine. Bring to the boil again, then remove from the heat and add the lemon zest and juice.

Serve the French toast topped with the compôte and, if you are feeling extra indulgent, with a spoonful of crème fraîche and a drizzle of maple syrup.

FOR THE VANILLA FRENCH TOAST:
4 eggs ....
250ml/9fl oz/1 cup full-fat milk ....
2 tbsp light soft brown sugar ....
2 tsp vanilla extract............................
¼ tsp sea salt ....
8 slices of stale Sharpham Park
    Farmhouse Loaf (see page 20)
    or other white spelt bread ....
1 tbsp sunflower oil ....
25g/1oz unsalted butter......................

FOR THE SUMMER BERRY
COMPÔTE:
500g/1lb 2oz mixed summer berries,
    such as raspberries, blueberries,
    cherries, blackberries, strawberries,
    redcurrants ....
80g/2¾oz/⅓ cup golden caster sugar,
    or more to taste...............................
grated zest and juice of 1 lemon ....
maple syrup, crème fraîche, Greek
    yogurt, Farmhouse Granola (see
    page 46) are all delicious optional
    extras ....

I remember, as a child, watching with fascination as my mother made pancakes. She made the most delicious pancakes, as she allowed time for the batter to rest, making it smooth and creamy. Raid your fridge and cupboards for fillings – a squeeze of lemon and a sprinkle of icing sugar, sliced bananas drizzled with clear honey, warmed blackcurrant jam, hazelnut and chocolate spread – whatever you feel like. Or take a look at our favourite serving suggestions, below.

BUTTERMILK PANCAKES

SERVES 4
PREPARATION TIME: 10 minutes, plus 1 hour resting COOKING TIME: 15 minutes

Sift the flour into a large bowl, add the salt and make a well in the centre. Add the eggs and whisk in gently. Gradually blend in the buttermilk, a little at a time, until the batter is smooth and the consistency of single cream.

Whisk 2 tablespoons of the melted butter into the mixture and reserve the rest of the butter for greasing the pan between pancakes. Leave the batter to rest for about 1 hour. This lets the starch cells in the spelt flour swell and creates a better pancake batter.

Heat the oven to its lowest setting. Grease a pancake or similar shallow frying pan with a little of the reserved butter, heat over the hob until hot, then carefully wipe away any excess butter with kitchen paper. Add a ladleful or 2 large spoonfuls of pancake batter to the pan and swirl it to form a circle. Cook for a few minutes until the edges start to brown, then flip the pancake over and cook the other side.

Transfer to the oven to keep the pancakes warm while you cook the rest, interleaving them with sheets of baking paper.

Serve with the topping of your choice (see right).

220g/7¾oz/1¾ cups white spelt flour
a pinch of sea salt ....
2 eggs, beaten ....
550ml/19fl oz/scant 2¼ cups
    buttermilk ....
55g/2oz unsalted butter, melted and
    cooled...

PANCAKE TOPPINGS

Be creative with your fillings and toppings, using these ideas or those suggested for Waffles (see page 61).

Savoury: sliced avocado, roasted tomatoes and chilli sauce; goat's cheese, beetroot and walnuts; melted cheese, toasted caraway seeds and creamed spinach.

Sweet: fresh seasonal berries; summer stone fruits, such as peaches and nectarines; poached rhubarb with Farmhouse Granola (see page 46); toasted nuts and/ or nut butters, such as almond, cashew or macadamia.

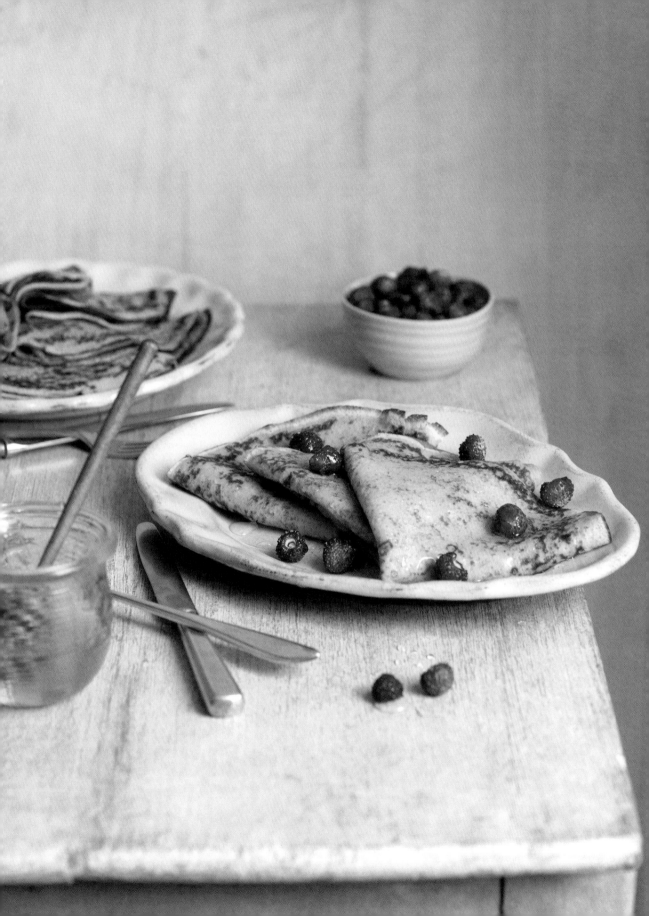

I always thought waffles were soft and served in piles, as they often are in the United States – until we tried making spelt ones for the Great British Spelt Recipe campaign. At our press launch we served savoury and sweet waffles, and I have never seen so many svelt and beautiful ladies demolish so many so fast! For this recipe, you will need a waffle iron. The easiest to use are the electric ones that you simply plug in – otherwise, they have to be heated on the hob. Experiment with the mouthwatering sweet and savoury toppings here, or devise your own creations.

WAFFLES

SERVES 4

PREPARATION TIME: 15 minutes, plus 45 minutes resting COOKING TIME: 20 minutes

Sift the dry ingredients together into a large bowl and make a well in the centre. In another smaller bowl, whisk together the eggs, milk, melted butter, vanilla and orange zest. Gradually pour the liquid ingredients into the well in the dry ingredients, whisking constantly, until all the ingredients are incorporated and you have a smooth batter. Cover and leave the batter to rest at room temperature for 30–45 minutes so that the spelt starch cells can swell. This makes for a better waffle batter.

Switch on the waffle iron and when it is hot, pour in a small ladleful of the batter, taking care not to overfill – an undersized waffle is better than a lava-like overspill. Close the waffle lid and cook until crisp – times will vary according to the type of machine you are using, but it should be about 3–5 minutes per waffle.

Serve with the topping of your choice.

300g/10½oz/2½ cups white
  spelt flour ....
2 tsp baking powder ....
4 tbsp caster sugar ....
a pinch of sea salt ....
1 tsp mixed spice ....
2 eggs ....
500ml/17fl oz/2 cups full-fat milk......
60g/2¼oz unsalted butter, melted and
  cooled..
2 tsp vanilla extract............................
grated zest of 1 large orange...............

SMOKED BACON & MAPLE SYRUP WAFFLES

Put half (or as many as will fit) the bacon rashers in a non-stick frying pan and fry over a medium heat for about 6 minutes, or until golden and crisp.

Remove from the heat and transfer to a plate lined with kitchen paper to absorb any excess fat. If necessary, keep them warm in the oven at 100°C/200°F/Gas ½ while you cook the the remaining bacon.

Pile the bacon on top of the waffles and drizzle with lots of maple syrup to serve.

12 smoked streaky bacon rashers ....
maple syrup, for drizzling ....

BANANA & CHOCOLATE HAZELNUT WAFFLES

Drizzle or smear the chocolate hazelnut spread over the waffles and put the banana slices on top, then scatter with the hazelnuts and cacao nibs, if using. Eat immediately.

200g/7oz good-quality chocolate
   hazelnut spread ....
2 bananas, sliced on the diagonal ....
100g/3½oz/¾ cup roasted, salted
   hazelnuts ....
50g/1¾oz/⅓ cup cocoa nibs
   (optional) ....

POACHED APRICOT WAFFLES

Put the fruit sugar in a saucepan over a medium heat with 500ml/17fl oz/2 cups water until all the sugar has dissolved, then add the vanilla, ginger and cardamom, stirring continuously. Add the apricots and bring to the boil, then turn the heat down to low and simmer for 10–15 minutes, or until they are soft. They shouldn't disintegrate into a mush, so don't stir too vigorously.

Remove the saucepan from the heat and add the lemon juice. Leave to cool slightly before serving on top of the waffles.

85g/3oz/⅓ cup fruit sugar ....
1 tsp vanilla extract ....
2.5cm/1in piece of root ginger, peeled
   and sliced into discs ....
seeds of 1 tbsp green cardamom pods,
   finely ground
500g/1lb 2oz apricots, halved and
   pitted ....
juice of ½ lemon ....

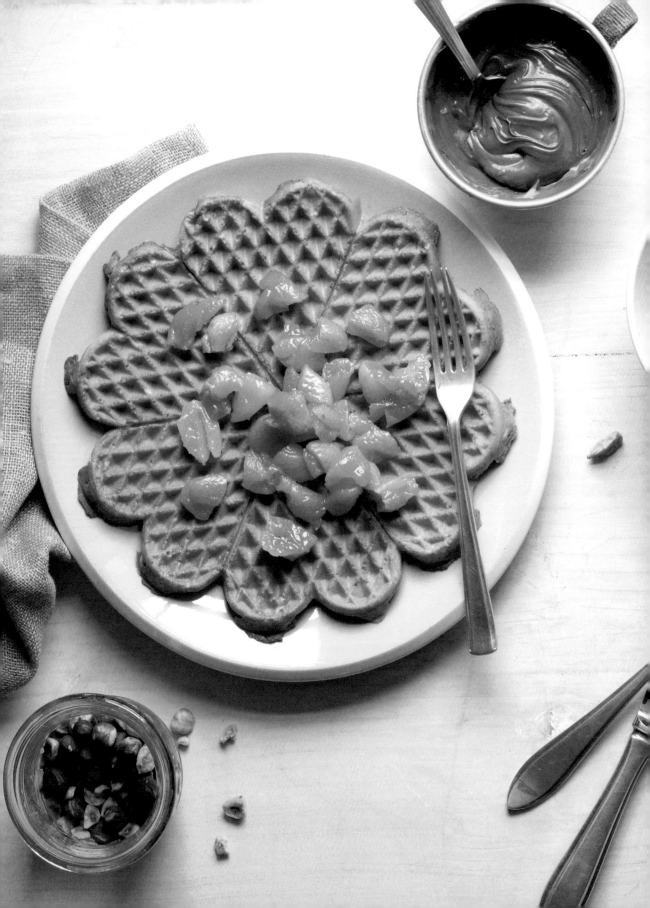

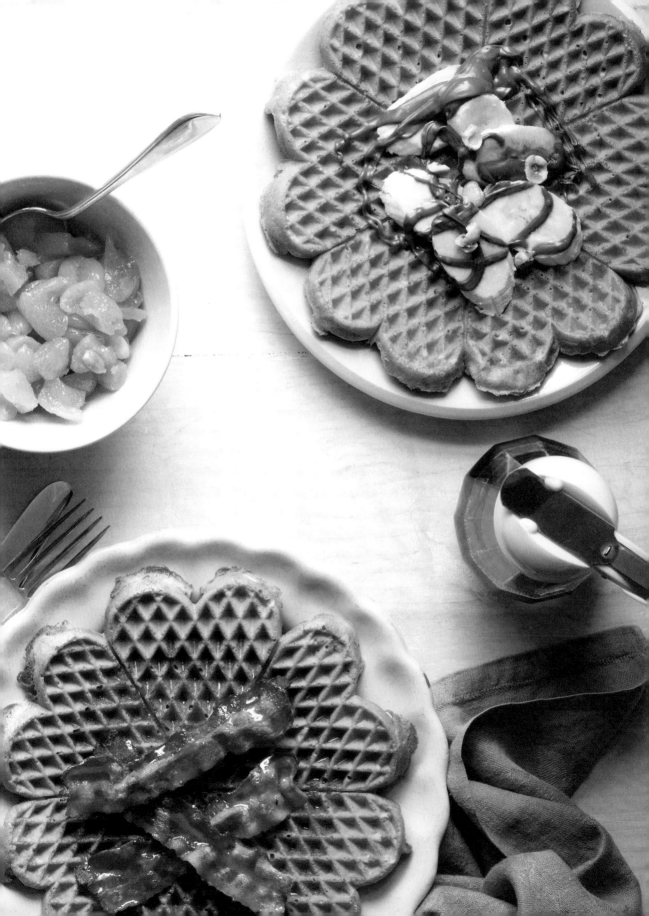

Spicy eggs are a modern breakfast or brunchtime favourite, and this version incorporates nutty pearled spelt to make a warming and nourishing start to your weekend. The green pepper in this recipe complements the chorizo and gives a sprightly freshness to the dish as a whole. You can obviously divide up the mixture into four individual earthenware dishes and bake the eggs in the oven, if you prefer, but the method we use is much more sociable.

SPICY SPANISH EGGS

SERVES 4
PREPARATION TIME: 20 minutes COOKING TIME: 45 minutes

Cook the pearled spelt in boiling water for 20 minutes, or until tender, following the packet instructions. Drain and leave to one side.

Heat the sunflower oil in a large, deep-sided sauté pan over a medium heat. Add the chorizo and cook for a few minutes until it caramelizes and starts to release its oil. Turn the slices over and cook on the other side for a couple of minutes. Remove from the pan, using a slotted spoon, transfer to a bowl and keep warm.

Add the onion, peppers and harissa paste to the pan and cook in the chorizo oil over a medium heat for about 10 minutes, stirring continuously with a wooden spoon until the vegetables are soft.

Add the garlic and cook for 1 minute. Add the tomatoes and stir well, then add 200ml/7fl oz/scant 1 cup water to the mixture so the tomatoes don't stick while cooking. Bring to the boil, then turn down the heat to medium and simmer for 15 minutes, or until the sauce has reduced and thickened.

Add the cooked pearled spelt and return the chorizo to the pan. Cook for a further 2–3 minutes, stirring, until all the ingredients are hot. Season with salt and pepper to taste.

Finally make 4 wells in the sauce mixture and crack an egg into each one. Cover the pan with a lid and poach the eggs for 5–8 minutes, or until they are set.

Serve the baked eggs in the dish you cooked them in, family style, scattered with the parsley and drizzled with a little olive oil. Let everyone garnish their own bowl with a lemon wedge and Greek yogurt, and serve with crusty bread, if you wish.

150g/5½oz/heaped ¾ cup pearled spelt...
1 tbsp sunflower oil ....
4 chorizo, about 300g/10½oz total weight, cut into 1cm/½in discs........
1 large Spanish onion, finely chopped
2 green peppers, deseeded and cut into 1cm/½in chunks ....
1 tbsp harissa paste ....
1 garlic clove, finely chopped.............
800g/1lb 12oz tinned plum tomatoes..
4 eggs ....
1 handful of parsley or coriander leaves, roughly shredded or chopped
a drizzle of olive oil...........................
sea salt and freshly ground black pepper ....
4 lemon wedges, to garnish................
4 tbsp Greek yogurt or labneh cheese, to garnish...........................
crusty bread, to serve (optional)..........

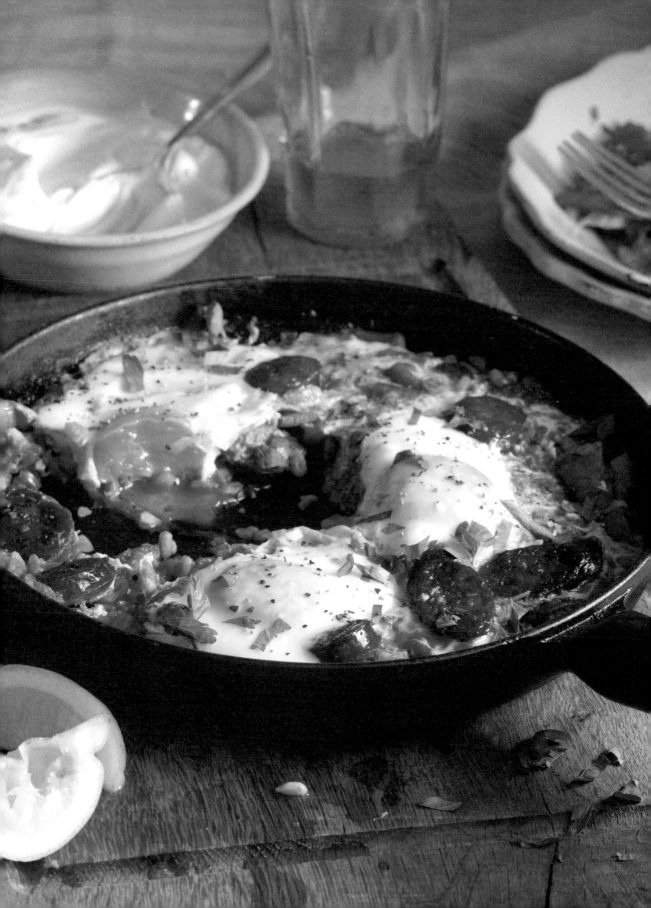

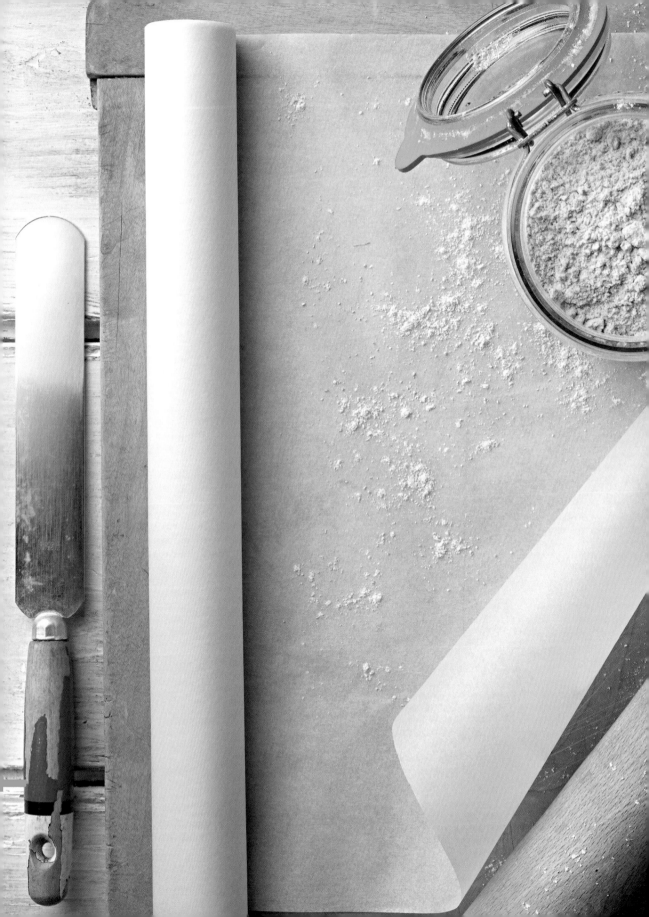

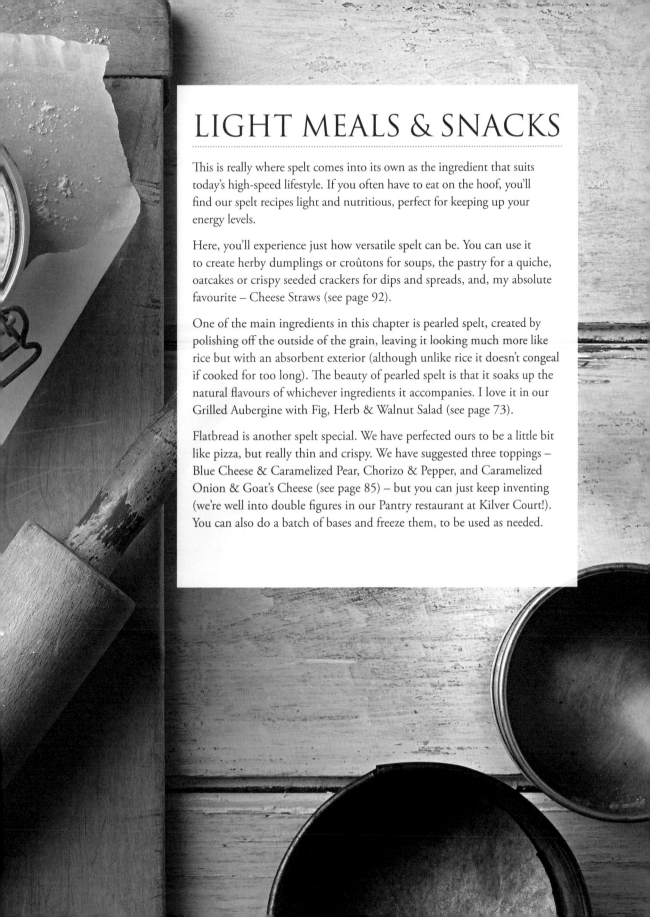

LIGHT MEALS & SNACKS

This is really where spelt comes into its own as the ingredient that suits today's high-speed lifestyle. If you often have to eat on the hoof, you'll find our spelt recipes light and nutritious, perfect for keeping up your energy levels.

Here, you'll experience just how versatile spelt can be. You can use it to create herby dumplings or croûtons for soups, the pastry for a quiche, oatcakes or crispy seeded crackers for dips and spreads, and, my absolute favourite – Cheese Straws (see page 92).

One of the main ingredients in this chapter is pearled spelt, created by polishing off the outside of the grain, leaving it looking much more like rice but with an absorbent exterior (although unlike rice it doesn't congeal if cooked for too long). The beauty of pearled spelt is that it soaks up the natural flavours of whichever ingredients it accompanies. I love it in our Grilled Aubergine with Fig, Herb & Walnut Salad (see page 73).

Flatbread is another spelt special. We have perfected ours to be a little bit like pizza, but really thin and crispy. We have suggested three toppings – Blue Cheese & Caramelized Pear, Chorizo & Pepper, and Caramelized Onion & Goat's Cheese (see page 85) – but you can just keep inventing (we're well into double figures in our Pantry restaurant at Kilver Court!). You can also do a batch of bases and freeze them, to be used as needed.

Nothing nourishes an ailing body quite like home-made chicken soup. Using roasted or barbecued bones adds much more flavour to this soup than if you use a raw chicken carcass, so it's well worth saving the bones left over from a Sunday roast chicken or if you do some barbecuing when the weather is balmy.

CHICKEN SOUP WITH SPELT & HERB DUMPLINGS

SERVES 4

PREPARATION TIME: **20 minutes** COOKING TIME: **1¾ hours**

Put the carrots, celery, onion, peppercorns, thyme, bayleaf and chicken carcass in a large saucepan and cover with cold water. Bring to the boil over a high heat, then turn the heat down to low and simmer gently for 1½ hours. Drain the broth into a clean saucepan, discarding the carcass, vegetables, peppercorns and herbs, then put the broth back on the hob and bring to a gentle simmer.

To make the herb dumplings, put the flours, Parmesan, baking powder, sea salt and chives in a large bowl, stir together and make a well in the centre. Add the buttermilk and egg and whisk until you have a thick, sticky dough, then stop. If you overmix, the dumplings will be tough. Shape the dough into dumplings using 2 tablespoons dipped in hot water and place the dumplings in the simmering broth. Add the chicken meat stripped from the carcass and wings and whichever fresh vegetables you wish. Cook for 5–10 minutes until the vegetables are tender, then serve the soup hot, garnished with herb sprigs.

FOR THE SOUP:

2 carrots, chopped ....

2 celery sticks, chopped ....

1 red onion, chopped ....

8 whole black peppercorns ....

1 bunch of thyme ....

1 bay leaf ....

1 roasted or cooked chicken carcass,
   meat stripped and reserved for the
   soup ....

8 roast or barbecued chicken wings ....

fresh vegetables, such as peas, fennel,
   kale, sweet potato, cabbage,
   broccoli, to serve ....

a few herbs sprigs, such as fennel,
   to serve ....

FOR THE DUMPLINGS:

125g/4½oz/1 cup white spelt flour

125g/4½oz/1 cup wholegrain spelt
   flour ....

55g/2oz/heaped ½ cup finely grated
   Parmesan cheese ....

2 tsp baking powder ....

½ tsp sea salt ....

1 bunch of chives, finely snipped ....

125ml/4 fl oz/½ cup buttermilk ....

1 egg ....

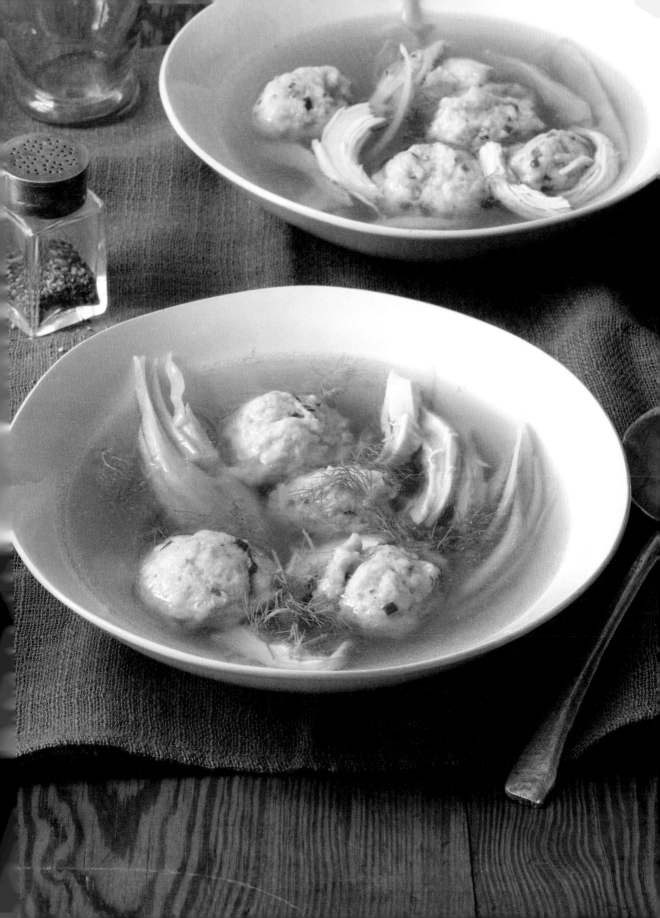

As the cooler days of autumn roll in, it's time to serve a big bowl of pumpkin soup, with these crisp spelt croûtons adding just the right amount of crunch to a simple lunch. You can use a chicken stock, or a vegetable stock if you are making a vegetarian version.

SPICED PUMPKIN SOUP WITH CROÛTONS

SERVES 4
PREPARATION TIME: 25 minutes COOKING TIME: 1¼ hours

Preheat the oven to 180°C/350°F/Gas 4.

Peel, deseed and chop the pumpkin into chunks and scatter the chunks of flesh in a large roasting dish or baking tray. Drizzle with a little oil and season with salt and pepper. Roast in the oven for 45 minutes, or until the pumpkin is soft and has taken on a little caramelized colour.

Meanwhile, heat 1 tablespoon olive oil in a large saucepan over a low heat and fry the onions for about 8 minutes, or until soft. Add the garlic and cook for a further minute, then add the allspice and cayenne and stir well. Add the roasted pumpkin, followed by the stock, sweet chilli sauce and vinegar. Bring to the boil, then turn the heat down to low and simmer for 30 minutes.

Once the pumpkin is cooked, turn the oven down to 150°C/300°F/Gas 2. Scatter the bread onto a baking sheet, drizzle with a little olive oil and season with salt and pepper. Bake for 30 minutes, or until the croûtons are dried out and very crisp. Remove from the oven and leave to cool.

Using a hand-held blender, carefully pulse the pumpkin soup until it is completely smooth. Taste and adjust the seasoning, if necessary, with more salt and pepper. Serve in individual bowls with a drizzle of olive oil, a scattering of pumpkin seeds and the spelt croûtons.

1 small pumpkin or butternut squash.
a little olive oil....................................
1 Spanish onion, finely chopped.........
1 garlic clove, finely chopped..............
4 allspice berries, finely crushed..........
a pinch of cayenne pepper ....
1 litre/35fl oz/4 cups chicken or
   vegetable stock.................................
1 tbsp sweet chilli or sriracha sauce.....
1 tsp balsamic vinegar........................
½ loaf of stale Ciabatta (see page 28)
   or Sharpham Park Farmhouse Loaf
   (see page 20), cut into 2cm/1in
   cubes ....
1 handful of pumpkin seeds ....
sea salt and freshly ground black
   pepper ....

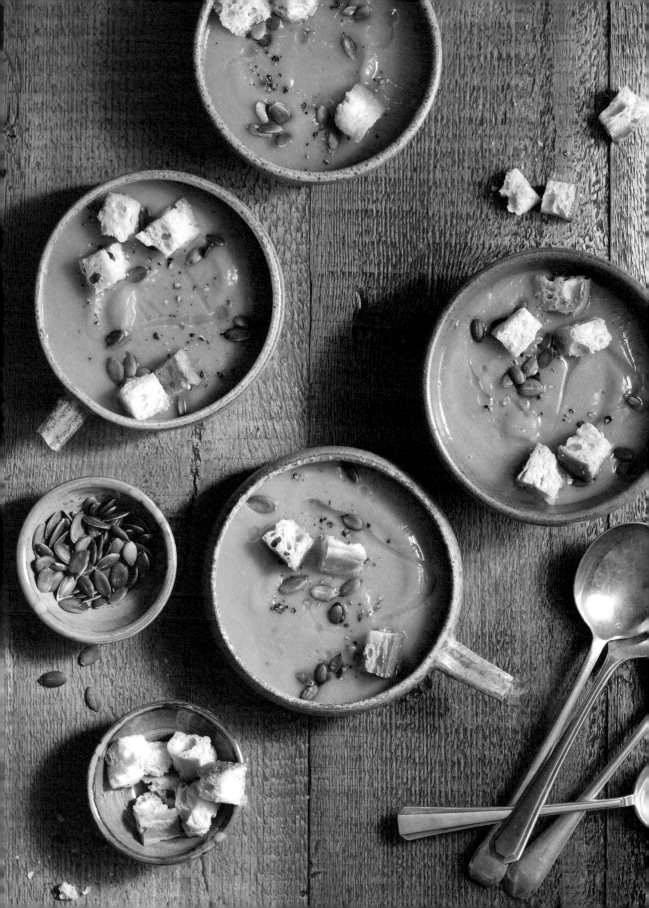

Green is the colour of spring, and this nutritious soup has plenty of green colour to go with its rich flavour – plus it's given extra crunch thanks to the crisply toasted spelt flakes scattered over the top.

PEA & SPRING GREEN SOUP WITH SPELT FLAKES

SERVES 4
PREPARATION TIME: 15 minutes COOKING TIME: 20 minutes

Warm the oil in a large saucepan over a low heat. Add the shallots and fry for 3–5 minutes until they are soft and translucent, without letting them brown. Add the garlic and fry for a further 30 seconds until the garlic loses its rawness, then add the peas, watercress and spring greens and stir well. Pour in the stock and bring to the boil, then turn down the heat to low and simmer gently for 10 minutes, or until the vegetables are tender.

Remove the pan from the heat and blend the soup, while it is still warm, using a hand-held blender. Do this slowly until all the soup is smooth. Season to taste with salt and pepper and add the vinegar to spruce up the flavour of the soup.

Scatter the spelt porridge flakes over the top and serve the warm soup immediately, sprinkled with pea shoots, a dash of Tabasco and a drizzle of oil, if you like.

2 tbsp sunflower oil ....
2 shallots, finely chopped ....
1 garlic clove, finely chopped.............
400g/14oz/2⅔ cups frozen or
    fresh podded peas ....
100g/3½oz watercress, washed ....
100g/3½oz spring greens, washed
    and chopped...................................
1 litre/35fl oz/4 cups vegetable
    or chicken stock...............................
½ tsp white wine vinegar or lemon
    juice..
1 small handful of spelt porridge
    flakes, lightly toasted.......................
sea salt and freshly ground white
    pepper ....
pea shoots, Tabasco sauce and olive or
    rapeseed oil, to serve (optional)........

This makes a great light meal on its own or as an accompaniment to grilled meat such as lamb, chicken or beef. The variety of contrasting textures makes it particularly interesting, with the soft aubergine, crunchy walnuts and luscious figs.

GRILLED AUBERGINE WITH FIG, HERB & WALNUT SALAD

SERVES 4
PREPARATION TIME: 20 minutes COOKING TIME: 15 minutes

Preheat the grill to medium-high.

Cut the aubergine into 1cm/½in thick discs and scatter them over a large rack that will fit under your grill (you may need to do this in batches). Brush with a little olive oil, then season with salt and pepper. Grill for a few minutes until the first side starts to go golden brown, then turn the aubergine slices over, brush with more olive oil, season again, then grill the other side until golden brown. This should take about 15 minutes in total, depending on how hot your grill is. Remove the aubergines from the heat and leave to one side.

Meanwhile, cook the pearled spelt in boiling water for 20 minutes, or until tender, following the packet instructions. Drain.

Make the dressing by whisking together the olive oil, lemon zest and juice and mustard in a large bowl, either by hand or using a hand-held blender. Add the herbs and capers and whisk again. Reserve about 3 tablespoons of the dressing to garnish. Pour the remainder over the cooked pearled spelt and toss together.

On a large serving plate or individual plates, start layering the ingredients in whichever order you choose. I start with aubergines, then figs. If they're not terribly sweet, you can add a drizzle of acacia blossom honey to the figs to bring out their flavour. Add the crumbled feta and dressed spelt, then finally add the toasted walnuts and drizzle the reserved dressing over the top. Finish with some extra parsley and mint leaves and serve at once.

2 large aubergines...............................
a drizzle of olive oil..............................
100g/3½oz/heaped ½ cup pearled
   spelt...
4 ripe figs, quartered or sliced............
a drizzle of clear acacia blossom honey
   (optional) ....
200g/7oz feta cheese, crumbled..........
150g/5½oz/scant 1¼ cups walnuts,
   lightly toasted ....
sea salt and freshly ground black
   pepper ....

FOR THE HERB DRESSING:
150ml/5fl oz/scant ⅔ cup olive oil .....
grated zest and juice of 1 large lemon .
1 tsp Dijon mustard ....
1 small bunch of parsley, finely
   chopped, plus extra to garnish ....
1 small bunch of mint, finely
   chopped, plus extra to garnish ....
1 tbsp capers, rinsed and drained........

This unusual and stunning summer salad was created by Scandinavian food writer Signe Johansen and is a riot of vibrant colours, textures and flavours. If you can't find wild dill pollen in your local delicatessen, you can buy small bottles online or simply leave it out.

BEETROOT, GOAT'S CURD, HAZELNUT & DILL SALAD

SERVES 4–6 as a main course
PREPARATION TIME: 20 minutes COOKING TIME: 45 minutes

Preheat the oven to 200°C/400°F/Gas 6.

Scrub the beetroot and trim off any gnarly bits. Put the beetroot in a roasting tin and pour in enough hot water to come halfway up the beetroot. Season generously with salt and pepper, then cover the tin with kitchen foil, sealing it tightly around the edges. Cook in the oven for 20 minutes for small beetroots and 40 minutes for really large ones.

Remove the tin from the oven and, using oven mitts, carefully lift the foil, keeping your hands and face away from the steam. Turn the beetroot over so that they cook evenly, then re-cover and cook for a further 20 or 40 minutes, as above, until tender.

Meanwhile, cook the pearled spelt in boiling water for 20 minutes, or until tender, following the packet instructions. Drain.

Remove the beetroot from the oven and leave to cool slightly, then drain off the cooking liquid. Peel off the skins while still warm. Cut the beetroot into quarters and put in a bowl. Pour over the raspberry vinegar and lemon juice to taste, then leave to one side. The beetroot is added last so that the dish doesn't turn entirely pink.

Toast the hazelnuts in a dry frying pan over a medium heat for a few minutes until golden and fragrant. Roll the nuts in a clean tea towel to remove the skins. Season with a little salt and crush into pieces.

Scatter the cooked spelt on a large serving plate and sprinkle with the wild dill pollen. Lift the beetroot out of the raspberry vinegar using a slotted spoon and put on top of the spelt, then scatter with the salad leaves, goat's curd and hazelnuts. Drizzle the vinegar over the top, if you like, or serve separately.

1.5kg/3lb 5oz beetroot ....
250g/9oz/heaped 1½ cups pearled spelt...
150ml/5fl oz/scant ⅔ cup raspberry vinegar...
juice of 2 lemons ....
4 tbsp hazelnuts, skin on ....
1 tsp wild dill pollen (optional) ....
200g/7oz seasonal salad leaves with edible flowers.................................
300g/10½oz goat's curd, crumbled.....
sea salt and freshly ground black pepper ....

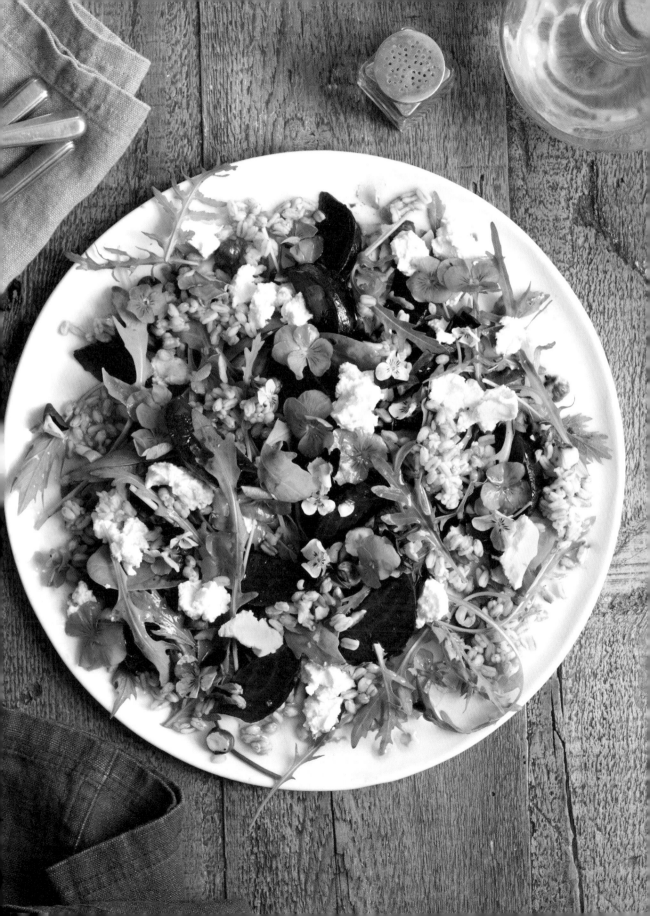

Almost one of the first spelt dishes we experimented with was a spelt crust quiche. These tarts were originally a German creation, although today we all know them by their French name 'quiche'. You can make so many different variations of this particular recipe and it is definitely one of my light-meal summer favourites served hot or cold.

BROCCOLI & COURGETTE QUICHE

MAKES 23cm/9in quiche
PREPARATION TIME: 20 minutes, plus making the pastry case and 20 minutes cooling
COOKING TIME: 25 minutes

Preheat the oven to 160°C/315°F/Gas 2–3 and grease a 23cm/9in flan dish.

Make the pastry, use to line the prepared dish and bake blind (see page 14). Sit the tin on a wire rack and leave to cool completely.

Bring a large saucepan of water to the boil and blanch the broccoli and courgettes for 1 minute, then drain and scatter across the cooled pastry case.

Whisk together the eggs and cream in a large bowl and season generously with nutmeg, salt and pepper. Pour this custard mixture over the vegetables and sprinkle the cheese and thyme leaves over the top.

Bake for 25 minutes, or until the quiche is set in the centre, then transfer to a wire rack to cool completely. Slice and serve with rocket salad, if you like.

1 recipe quantity Shortcrust Pastry (see page 14) ....
200g/7oz broccoli, cut into small florets ....
2 small courgettes, coarsely grated ......
6 eggs ....
200ml/7fl oz/scant 1 cup double cream..
½ tsp freshly grated nutmeg, or to taste ....
100g/3½oz/¾ cup blue cheese, grated
leaves from 1 large thyme sprig...........
sea salt and freshly ground black pepper ....
rocket salad, to serve (optional) ....

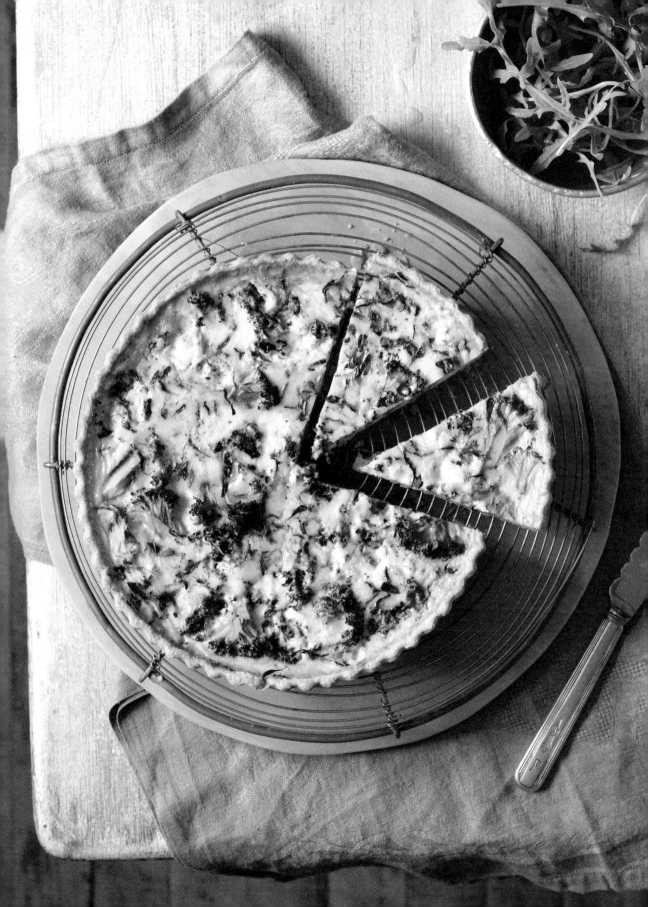

The Italians have ingenious ways of reinventing leftovers and this is no exception. Arancini are traditionally made with leftover rice and seasoned with any number of delicious flavours, such as cheese, ragu, sun-dried tomatoes or a mixture of herbs and vegetables. Here we have used spelt in place of the rice. They make a great snack at a party or, if you're not feeling terribly inspired by the thought of sandwiches for lunch, here is your perfect solution.

ARANCINI

SERVES 4–6 as a generous snack
PREPARATION TIME: 25 minutes, plus making the speltotto COOKING TIME: 30 minutes

Divide the speltotto mixture into 16 balls and flatten them in your palm or on a clean work surface. Place the small mozzarella ball in the centre and fold up the speltotto mixture around the ball of cheese.

Line up three bowls, one with the flour, the next with the eggs and the third with the breadcrumbs, and line a baking sheet with baking paper. Heat the oil in a deep-fat fryer or in a large, heavy-based saucepan to 160°C/315°F. Meanwhile, dust each arancini ball with a light coating of flour, then dip in the egg and finally roll in the panko breadcrumbs. Put them all on the prepared baking sheet.

When the oil is hot, fry a few at a time, making sure the oil doesn't dip much below 160°C/315°F or go too high. Cook each batch of arancini for a minute or so and then turn them over, if necessary, to cook the other side. Remove with a slotted spoon and put them on a plate lined with kitchen paper to absorb the excess oil. Repeat the process with the remaining arancini. Serve warm or cold, on their own or with a fresh green salad, if you like.

½ recipe quantity Wild Mushroom
   & Roast Chicken Speltotto
   (see page 137) ....
16–20 small balls of mozzarella
   cheese ....
a little white spelt flour, for dusting ....
2 eggs, lightly beaten ....
a small bowl of panko breadcrumbs....
sunflower oil, for deep-frying ....
fresh green salad, to serve
   (optional) ....

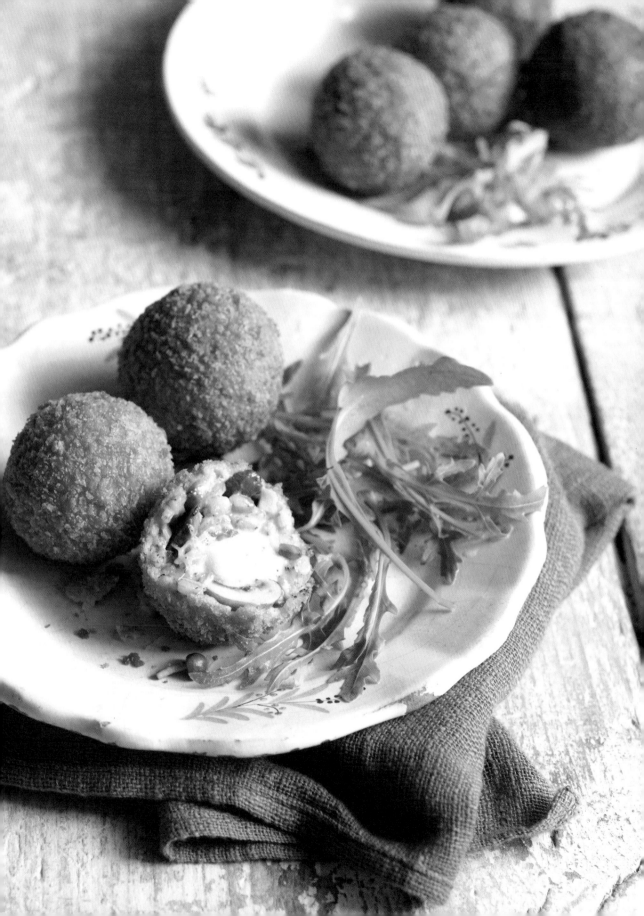

Couscous is originally a Berber dish from North Africa. At first it was made from millet, but that was gradually replaced by wheat in the 20th century. This vibrant, colourful spelt couscous dish is ideal for lazy summer days when you don't want to slave over a stove in the kitchen. It's quick to prepare and requires minimal effort, just assemble it up to half an hour before you plan on serving it and watch as those around you go 'Wow!' and make appreciative noises!

COUSCOUS WITH PROSCIUTTO, PEACHES & BURRATA

SERVES: 4
PREPARATION TIME: 20 minutes

Put the spelt couscous in a large bowl and pour over the hot stock. Stir well, then cover with a plate and allow the couscous to swell for a few minutes.

Next, take a fork and run it through the couscous so that it fluffs up. Drizzle with olive oil and keep fluffing until you have no more large lumps of soaked couscous left.

Spread the couscous over a large serving plate, or individual plates, then sprinkle the burrata on top, then the prosciutto, peaches and tomatoes. Scatter the basil leaves and pine nuts over the top, drizzle with a little olive oil and balsamic vinegar, and season with a little salt and pepper to taste.

200g/7oz/scant 1 cup spelt couscous ....
400ml/14fl oz/generous 1½ cups boiling hot vegetable stock..............
a drizzle of olive oil............................
2 x 200g/7oz balls of burrata cheese, shredded ....
150g/5½oz prosciutto, sliced.............
4 ripe peaches, pitted and cut into 8...
4 ripe tomatoes, preferably Marinda or beefsteak, cut into 8 ....
1 handful of basil leaves......................
1 handful of toasted pine nuts ....
a drizzle of balsamic vinegar
sea salt and freshly ground black pepper ....

A healthy sandwich wrap full of Northern European flavours, this makes a great lunch or light meal and takes only minutes to prepare. The sharpness of the lemon and the fiery horseradish crème offer a perfect complement to the other ingredients.

SMOKED SALMON WRAPS WITH BEETROOT, DILL & HORSERADISH

SERVES 4

PREPARATION TIME: 10 minutes, plus 1 hour resting COOKING TIME: 15 minutes

Mix together all the ingredients for the wraps with 150ml/5fl oz/scant ⅔ cup warm water in a large bowl to make a soft dough, and knead lightly for a few minutes until it is smooth and no longer sticky, adding a little extra water if the dough appears too dry. Cover with a clean, damp tea towel and leave to rest for 1 hour.

Turn the dough out onto a lightly floured work surface and divide into quarters. Roll them out as thinly as possible into circles about 23cm/9in in diameter.

Heat a little oil in a large sauté pan and fry the wraps, individually if necessary, for about 2 minutes on each side until golden brown. Remove them from the pan and wrap in a clean tea towel until you are ready to use them, so that they stay soft. Leave to cool.

Spread the spelt wraps on a work surface and divide the smoked salmon equally among them.

Put the crème fraîche, dill, horseradish sauce and lemon zest and juice in a bowl. Season with pepper and add more lemon juice if you like a strong lemon flavour.

Spread the crème fraîche mixture over the salmon, then add the sliced beetroot and scatter some salad leaves on top before folding up the wraps and eating immediately.

FOR THE SPELT WRAPS:
2 tsp olive oil, plus extra for frying .....
125g/4½oz/1 cup white spelt flour, plus extra for dusting ....
125g/4½oz/1 cup wholegrain spelt flour ....
½ tsp sea salt ....

FOR THE SMOKED SALMON & BEETROOT FILLING:
400g/14oz smoked salmon ....
200g/7oz/scant 1 cup crème fraîche....
1 small bunch of dill, chopped ....
2 tbsp strong horseradish sauce...........
grated zest and juice of ½ lemon, or to taste...
freshly ground black pepper ....
200g/7oz pickled beetroot, sliced ....
salad leaves of your choice, such as watercress, spinach, rocket ....

This cornbread is best eaten slightly warm, and is utterly delicious on its own or with the Spiced Beef Hot Pot (see page 130), with a soup, such as the Spiced Pumpkin Soup with Croûtons (see page 70) or with a bowl of warming chilli con carne. It's a doddle to make and is a real crowd pleaser. If you're not a fan of feta, try this with some strong Cheddar, roughly grated, or some Parmesan.

FETA & JALAPEÑO CORNBREAD

MAKES 20 x 30cm/12 x 8in cornbread
PREPARATION TIME: 20 minutes COOKING TIME: 30 minutes

Preheat the oven to 220°C/425°F/Gas 7. Lightly oil a 30 x 20cm/ 12 x 8in baking tin.

Put all the dry ingredients in a large bowl, stir together and make a well in the centre. Add the eggs, buttermilk and honey and fold everything together, working quite quickly as the liquid activates the raising agents, until the mixture is smooth (there can be a lump or two of dry ingredients bobbing around).

Fold in the jalapeños and the feta cheese. Stir through a few more times and then pour the cornbread mixture into the prepared tin.

Bake for 30 minutes, or until the top is golden brown and a skewer inserted in the centre comes out clean. Transfer the cornbread to a wire rack to cool. Cut into squares to serve.

a little oil, for greasing ....
250g/9oz/1⅔ cups cornmeal ....
250g/9oz/2 cups white spelt flour.......
2½ tsp baking powder........................
¼ tsp bicarbonate of soda...................
½ tsp sea salt ....
¼ tsp freshly ground black pepper......
3 eggs, lightly beaten ....
250ml/9fl oz/1 cup buttermilk...........
2 tbsp clear honey ....
100g/3½oz jalapeño peppers, drained
   of their preserving liquid.................
100g/3½oz feta cheese, diced ....

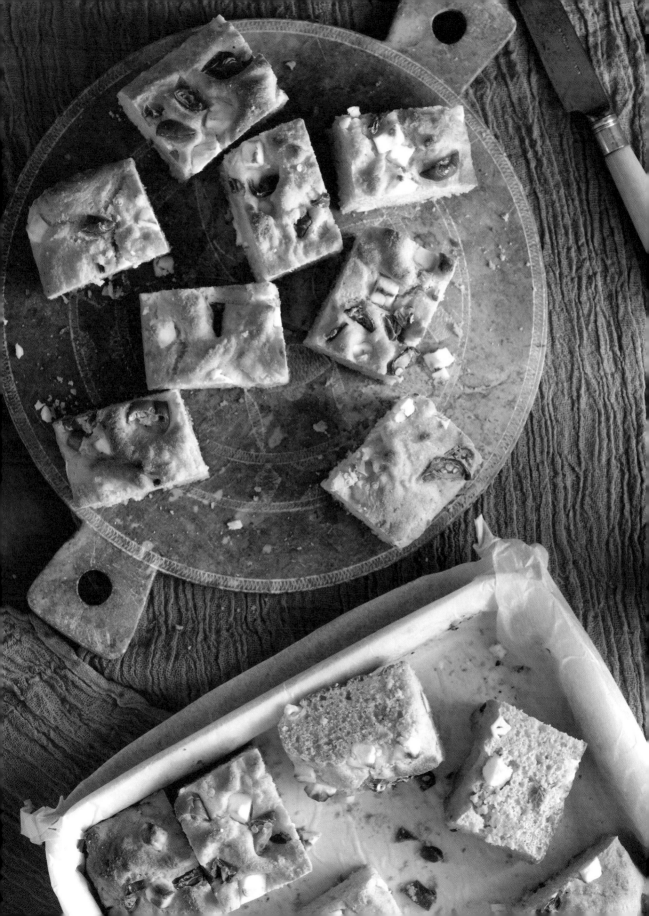

This nutty flatbread recipe was created by our local baker, Lievito, who makes these for our restaurant at Kilver Court in Somerset. You can also make it with half white and half wholegrain spelt flour. Here are three different toppings for our flatbreads, but do experiment to your heart's content. We just keep adding new ones in our restaurant!

FLATBREADS

MAKES 4 x 15 x 25cm/6 x 10in flatbreads
PREPARATION TIME: 30 minutes, plus 1 hour resting COOKING TIME: 10 minutes

Lightly oil two large baking sheets.

Mix together all the ingredients with 150ml/5fl oz/scant ⅔ cup water in a large bowl to make a soft dough, and knead lightly for a few minutes until it is smooth and no longer sticky. Cover with a clean, damp tea towel and leave to rest for 1 hour.

Preheat the oven to 200°C/400°F/Gas 6.

Turn the dough out onto a lightly floured surface and divide into four equal pieces. Roll them out as thinly as possible to about 15 x 25cm/ 6 x 10in and put on the prepared baking sheets. Bake for 10 minutes until just browned.

Remove from the oven and continue with your chosen topping.

2 tsp olive oil, plus extra
   for greasing.....................................
250g/9oz/2 cups white spelt flour,
   plus extra for dusting......................
½ tsp sea salt ....

BLUE CHEESE & CARAMELIZED PEAR FLATBREADS

Sprinkle the cheese over the flatbreads and leave to one side while you caramelize the pears. Slice the pears into quarters (or eighths if very big) and remove the cores.

Melt the butter and sugar together in a large frying pan over a medium heat until foaming slightly, then add the pears. Cook on each side for a couple of minutes, or until the pear lightly caramelizes.

Remove the pears from the pan and distribute between the flatbreads. Scatter the walnuts on the top and heat in the oven for 5–10 minutes to allow the cheese to melt slightly. Serve hot.

200g/7oz blue cheese of choice, crumbled or diced..........................
4 small pears..
55g/2oz unsalted butter.....................
60g/2¼oz/⅓ cup light soft brown sugar...
1 handful of walnuts..........................

CHORIZO & PEPPER FLATBREADS

Heat the oil in a large frying pan over a medium heat, add the chorizo and fry for a few minutes until lightly browned and the oil starts to leach out of the sausages. Using a slotted spoon, remove the chorizo from the pan and leave to one side.

Add the peppers to the pan and fry for 5 minutes until they start to soften. Add the onion and cook for a further 5–10 minutes until the peppers are soft and the onion is translucent and soft.

Return the chorizo to the pan and warm through for a minute, then add the lemon zest and juice (you can use more if you like a citrus kick from the lemon), then scatter the parsley on top and stir through again. Scoop spoonfuls of the topping onto the warmed flatbreads, drizzle with olive oil and serve hot.

2 tbsp olive oil, plus extra for drizzling...
4 hot chorizo sausages, sliced into discs...
1 red pepper, deseeded and sliced ....
1 green pepper, deseeded and sliced....
1 Spanish onion, finely chopped.........
grated zest and juice of ½ lemon, or to taste...
1 handful of parsley leaves, chopped...

CARAMELIZED ONION & GOAT'S CHEESE FLATBREADS

Heat the oil in a large frying pan and fry onions for 15 minutes, or until soft. Add the sugar and stir until all the sugar has dissolved. Season with the balsamic vinegar.

Preheat the grill to medium.

Spoon the onion mixture over the tops the flatbreads. Put 4 discs of goat's cheese on top of each one, then grill for 3–5 minutes, until just melted and golden, then serve warm with a few salad leaves.

2 tbsp sunflower oil ....
4 small red onions, finely chopped .....
55g/2oz/scant ⅓ cup dark soft brown sugar..
2 tbsp balsamic vinegar......................
24 discs of goat's cheese ....
mixed leaves of your choice, to serve...

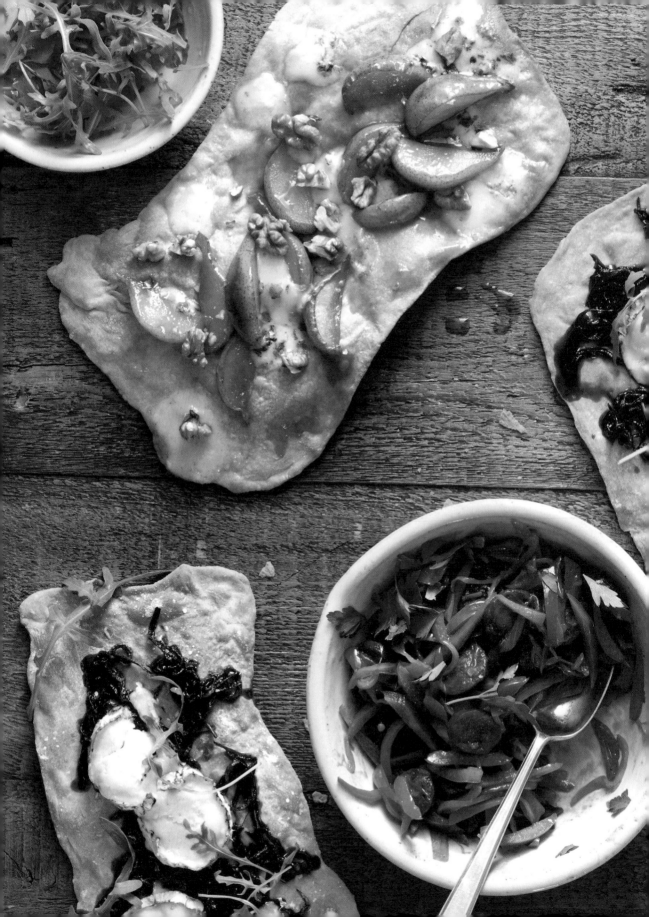

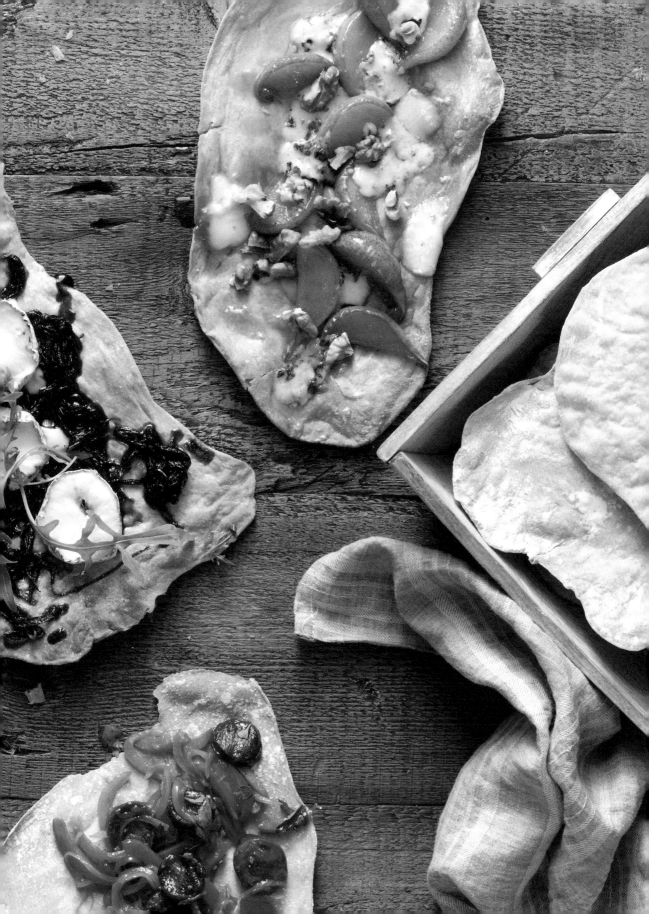

Crisp, crunchy crackers with seeds are always a good standby when you're entertaining, and these taste so much better than the ones you find in a store. I could eat these crackers all day, and paired with the mackerel dip, they make a perfect snack.

SEEDED CRACKERS WITH SMOKED MACKEREL DIP

MAKES 20 crackers
PREPARATION TIME: 10 minutes, plus 30 minutes chilling COOKING TIME: 5 minutes

Lightly oil a large bowl.

Put the flour, salt and baking powder in another large bowl, mix well and make a well in the centre. Add the oil and 125ml/4fl oz/½ cup ice-cold water. Mix together, using a wooden spoon, to a rough dough. Turn the dough out onto a lightly floured work surface and knead gently until smooth, then flatten into a disc. Transfer to the prepared bowl, cover with cling film and chill in the fridge for 30 minutes.

Preheat the oven to 200°C/400°F/Gas 6 and line a large baking sheet with baking paper.

Roll out the dough on a lightly floured work surface into a thin sheet (the thinner you roll out the dough, the crisper the crackers with be). Brush with oil and scatter the seeds on top, along with extra sea salt, if you wish. Cut into 20 rectangles or squares, or use a biscuit cutter if you want perfectly round or shaped crackers, then put them on the prepared baking sheet.

Bake for 3–5 minutes until the crackers are crisp, have risen and feel sandy to the touch. Transfer to a wire rack to cool.

Pulse all the dip ingredients in a blender until smooth. Season to taste with salt and pepper. Serve the crackers and dip, garnished with herbs, if you like.

FOR THE CRACKERS:
2 tbsp olive or rapeseed oil, plus extra for greasing and brushing.................
220g/8oz/1¾ cups white spelt flour, or equal quantities of white and wholegrain spelt flour, plus extra for dusting ....
¾ tsp fine sea salt, plus extra for brushing ....
¾ tsp baking powder ....
3 tbsp mixed seeds, such as flaxseed, poppy, chia, sesame........................

FOR THE SMOKED MACKEREL DIP:
2 skinless smoked mackerel fillets ....
200ml/7fl oz/scant 1 cup crème fraîche..
2 tbsp horseradish sauce ....
1 bunch of parsley or dill, plus extra, roughly chopped, to garnish ....
grated zest and juice of 1 lemon ....
a pinch of black pepper ....

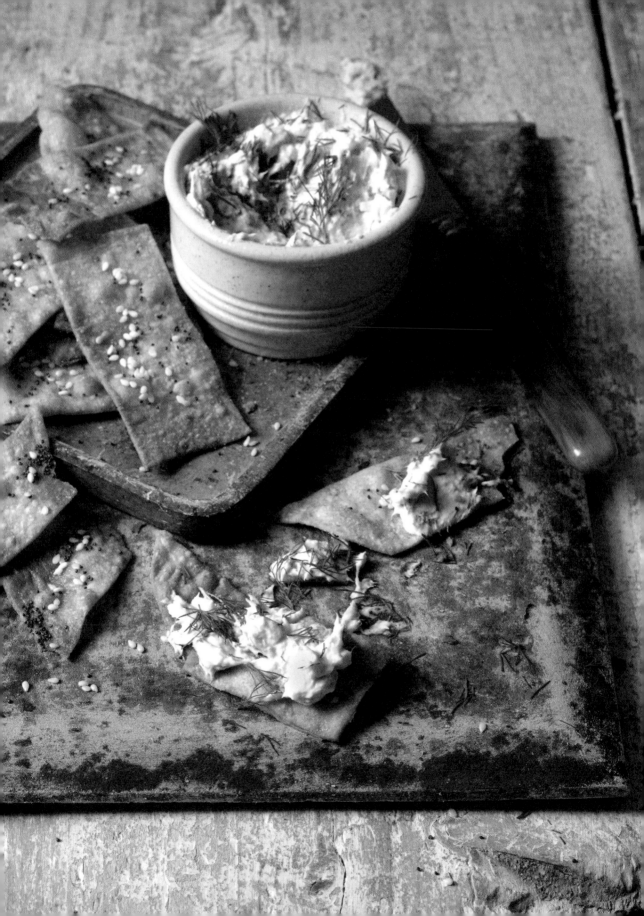

This recipe took a lot of experimentation. At first we tried to make it with 100% spelt, but found that adding some oats gave them that traditional flavour. They make delicious hors d'oeuvres with all sorts of savoury toppings – my favourite is mature Cheddar, chutney and chives – but they are equally at home with the cheese board.

OATCAKES

MAKES about 20 oatcakes
PREPARATION TIME: 25 minutes COOKING TIME: 25 minutes

Preheat the oven to 180°C/350°F/Gas 4 and lightly grease two baking sheets or line with baking paper.

Put all the ingredients in a large bowl, stir together and make a well in the centre. Add 115ml/3¾fl oz/scant ½ cup boiling water, stir through and leave the mixture to settle for about 10 minutes until it is at room temperature.

Sprinkle the extra ground spelt porridge flakes on a clean work surface. Divide the dough in half, then roll out each piece until the dough is 5mm/¼in thick. Use a cutter of your choice to cut out the oatcakes and put them on the prepared baking sheets.

Bake for 20–25 minutes, or until the oatcakes are pale golden in colour and feel sandy to the touch. Transfer to a wire rack to cool.

3 tbsp olive oil, plus extra for greasing (optional) ....
100g/3½oz/heaped ¾ cup oatmeal.....
55g/2oz/heaped ½ cup spelt porridge flakes, ground in a small blender or pestle and mortar, plus extra for dusting..
55g/2oz/scant ½ cup wholegrain spelt flour ....
½ tsp caster sugar ....
½ tsp salt...

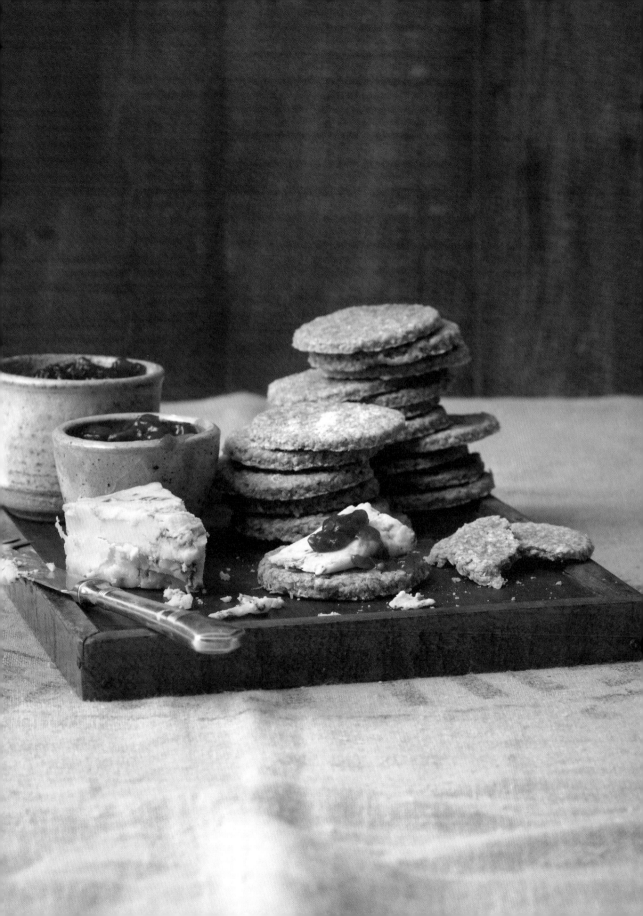

My first encounter with cheese straws was at aged five, pinching them, at full stretch, from my grandmother's dining table. They remain a favourite today, and we like to think we have improved on them by making them with spelt flour. Sorry, Granny!

CHEESE STRAWS

MAKES about 20
PREPARATION TIME: 20 minutes, plus 1 hour chilling COOKING TIME: 15 minutes

Preheat the oven to 190°C/375°F/Gas 5 and lightly grease a baking sheet or line with baking paper.

Put the flour and spices in a large bowl and rub in the butter and lard, using your fingertips, until the mixture resembles fine breadcrumbs. Add half the grated Cheddar and stir together, then add the egg and 1 tablespoon ice-cold water. Bring together, using a wooden spoon, adding a little more water if the mixture looks dry. Lightly knead the dough for a few seconds until smooth and there are no major lumps of dry mixture.

Shape the dough into a rectangle about 40 x 30cm/16 x 12in and cut into 1cm/½in slices. Put on the prepared baking sheets, cover with cling film and chill for 1 hour or until the straws are firm.

Sprinkle the extra grated cheese on top, then bake in the oven for 15 minutes, or until the biscuits are golden brown and feel sandy to the touch. Transfer to a wire rack to cool.

125g/4½oz cold unsalted butter, diced, plus extra for greasing (optional) ....
250g/9oz/2 cups white spelt flour, or half white and half wholegrain spelt flour ....
¼ tsp cayenne pepper ....
¼ tsp mustard powder......................
a pinch of freshly grated nutmeg ....
a pinch of freshly ground white pepper ....
55g/2oz cold lard, diced ....
150g/5½oz/1⅓ cups strong Cheddar cheese, finely grated, plus extra to garnish..............................
1 egg, beaten ....

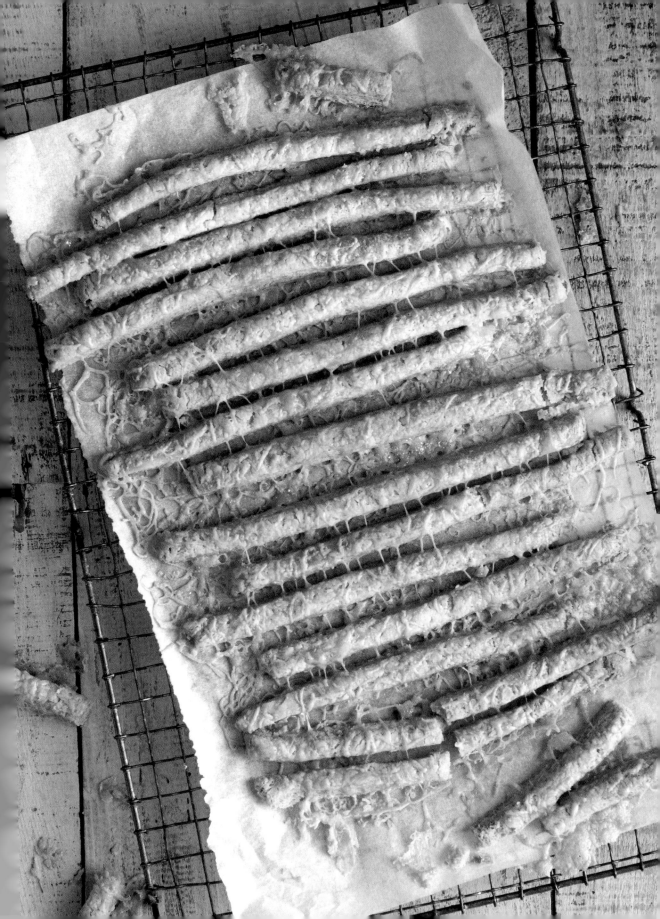

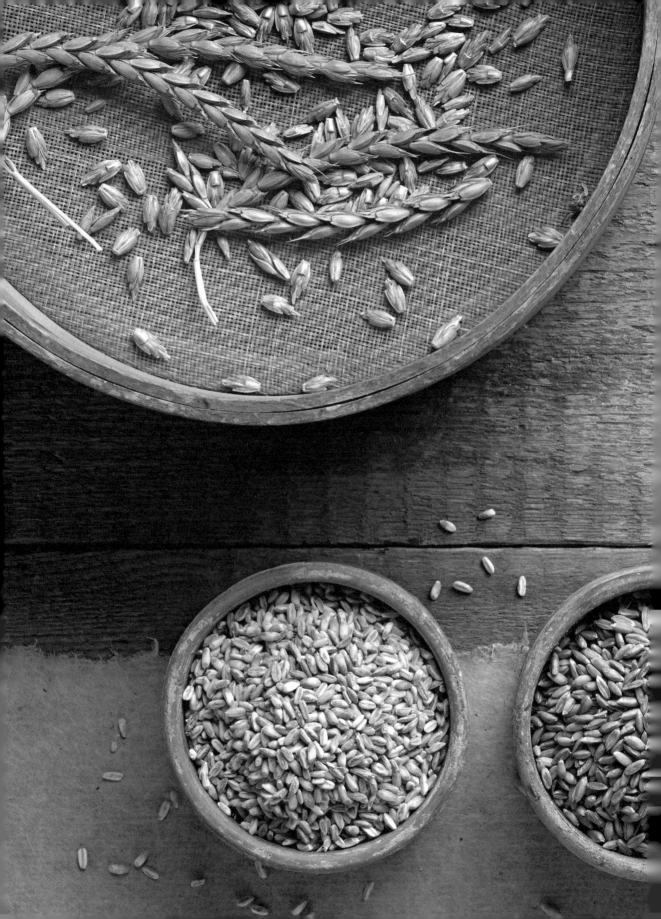

AFTERNOON TEA

Afternoon tea is a peculiarly British custom, but one that has become popular and is now practiced all over the world. As a meal, it didn't really appear until the mid 1800s, when the Duchess of Bedford created a fashion for it. At our Harlequin Cafe at Kilver Court in Somerset, we serve loose tea in a random selection of mismatched vintage china with the most scrumptuous spelt cakes on floral cake stands.

Cakes and pastry really showcase the lovely nuttiness of spelt, adding an extra dimension to the flavour. I love including walnuts or almonds to increase that nutty crunch. Walnuts have been a staple at Sharpham Park and the Glastonbury area for over 500 years, and we've planted 300 trees to continue the tradition. Here, the nuts help to create a spectacular Carrot Cake (see page 103), as well as the Walnut & Coffee Cake with Streusel Topping (see page 106). And I can never resist anything with almonds, whether it is our Plum & Frangipane Cake (see page 104) or the Summer Raspberry Cake (see page 108).

And once the summer and autumn fruits are no longer in season, you can enjoy our Mince Pies (see page 116) for a very festive Christmas treat.

As spelt is lower in gluten, you get a crunchier result when making cookies, plus you can vary the flavours almost infinitely, depending on the ingredients you have in the cupboard. So whether you go for white chocolate and cranberries, sultanas and orange zest, or date and cinnamon, you can mix and bake a batch of delicious fresh cookies in next to no time. Ring the changes, too, by using either spelt porridge flakes or spelt muesli, while a soft brown sugar will give you a different flavour from a golden caster sugar.

COOKIES

MAKES about 30 cookies
PREPARATION TIME: 20 minutes   COOKING TIME: 15 minutes

Start by making the cookie base. Put the spelt porridge flakes, flours and sugar in a large bowl.

Melt the butter and honey together in a heavy-based saucepan over a low heat. Add the bicarbonate of soda and vanilla and mix together.

Pour this mixture into the dry ingredients, then continue with your chosen cookie variation.

175g/6oz/1¾ cups spelt porridge flakes or Monty's Muesli (see page 48)...................................
55g/2oz/scant ½ cup white spelt flour, plus extra for dusting.............
55g/2oz/scant ½ cup wholegrain spelt flour ....
115g/4oz/½ cup golden caster sugar or light soft brown sugar.................
115g/4oz salted butter.......................
3 tbsp clear honey ....
1 tsp bicarbonate of soda...................
1 tsp vanilla extract............................

CHOCOLATE CHIP GRANOLA COOKIES

Preheat the oven to 180°C/350°F/Gas 4 and line two baking sheets with baking paper.

Mix the dough ingredients, using the muesli instead of spelt porridge flakes and light soft brown sugar instead of caster sugar. Add the chocolate chunks to the bowl and mix to a soft dough.

Shape into 30 balls, using lightly floured hands, then flatten into discs and put on the prepared baking sheets. Bake for 10–15 minutes until the biscuits are golden brown and firm around the edges.

Leave to cool on the baking sheets for 3 minutes, then transfer to a wire rack to cool completely.

115g/4oz/heaped 1 cup dark chocolate chunks ....

GINGER & HONEY COOKIES

Preheat the oven to 180°C/350°F/Gas 4 and line two baking sheets with baking paper.

Mix the dough ingredients, add the spice, if using, and ginger to the bowl and mix to a soft dough.

Shape into 30 balls, using lightly floured hands, then flatten into discs and put on the prepared baking sheets. Bake for 10–15 minutes until the biscuits are golden brown and firm around the edges.

Leave to cool on the baking sheets for 3 minutes, then transfer to a wire rack to cool completely.

1 tsp mixed spice, or spice of your choice (optional)............................
115g/4oz/½ cup stem ginger pieces, drained ....

FRUIT & NUT COOKIES

Preheat the oven to 180°C/350°F/Gas 4 and line two baking sheets with baking paper.

Mix the dough ingredients, add the fruit and nuts to the bowl and mix to a soft dough.

Shape into 30 balls, using lightly floured hands, then flatten into discs and put on the prepared baking sheets. Bake for 10–15 minutes until the biscuits are golden brown and firm around the edges.

Leave to cool on the baking sheets for 3 minutes, then transfer to a wire rack to cool completely.

75g/2½oz/⅔ cup mixed dried fruit, such as pitted and chopped dates and apricots, sultanas, sour cherries, cranberries...................
75g/2½oz/½ cup unsalted pistachios or mixed nuts such as almonds, macadamias, pecans, walnuts ....

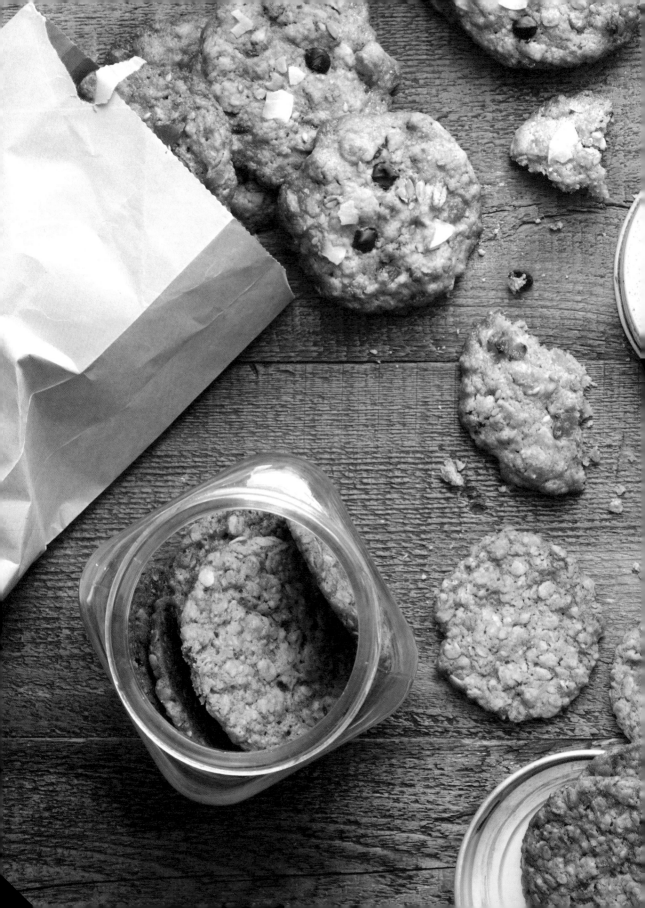

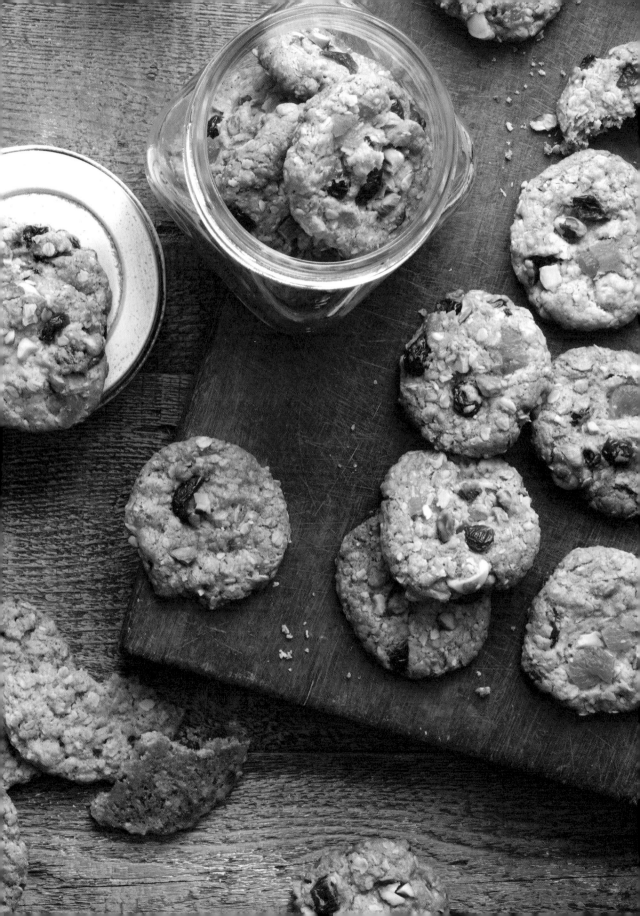

These are my favourite bite-sized nibble – perhaps because years of working in Italy buying leather and fabric for my Mulberry designs meant industrial quantities of biscotti dipped in vin santo! These light and aromatic biscotti are great for a tea-time snack, and you can vary the flavours – include spices, or try different nuts, such as walnuts, almonds or pecans.

PISTACHIO, LEMON & VANILLA BISCOTTI

MAKES about 40 biscotti
PREPARATION TIME: 30 minutes COOKING TIME: 1 hour

Preheat the oven to 180°C/350°F/Gas 4 and line two baking sheets with baking paper.

Beat together the butter, sugar and vanilla extract in a large bowl, using an electric mixer, until pale and fluffy. Add the eggs one at a time, including a spoonful of the flour with each egg to prevent the mixture from splitting. Mix the remaining flour with the baking powder, salt and lemon zest in a medium bowl. Add half to the egg mixture with half the lemon juice and blend together gently, then blend in enough of the remaining lemon juice to give you a soft dough. You may not need all the lemon juice as you do not want the dough to be too wet. Finally, mix in the toasted pistachios.

Turn the dough out onto a lightly floured work surface, divide into four equal-sized pieces and roll each one into a log about 25cm/10in long. Put the biscotti logs on the prepared baking sheets, spacing them at least 10cm/4in apart as they will spread when baking.

Bake them on the middle shelf of the oven for 25 minutes, or until they have risen, feel firm and look golden. Remove the logs from the oven, turn the heat down to 150°C/300°F/Gas 2 and transfer the biscotti logs to a wire rack to cool slightly, then cut them into 1cm/½in thick diagonal slices.

Put these back on the baking sheets, flat-side down, and return them to the oven for a further 15 minutes on each side until dried out. Transfer to a wire rack to cool. If they are still a little chewy, you can always pop the biscotti back in a preheated oven at 100°C/200°F/Gas ½ and dry them out for 30 minutes.

115g/4oz unsalted butter, softened .....
175g/6oz/¾ cup golden caster sugar ...
1 tsp vanilla extract ....
3 eggs ....
350g/12oz/2¾ cups white spelt
   flour ....
2½ tsp baking powder ....
¼ tsp salt ....
grated zest and juice of 1 small lemon
115g/4oz/¾ cup unsalted pistachios,
   lightly toasted ....

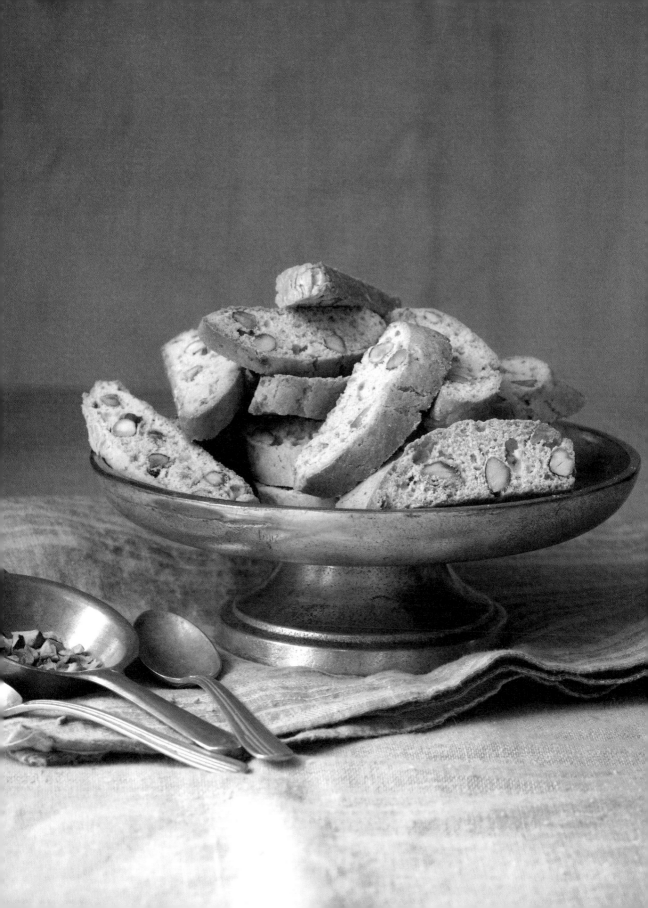

Edd Kimber, winner of the first series of the BBC's *The Great British Bake Off*, gave us these delectable chocolate sables to use in partnership with the Bowel Cancer Campaign of 2013. *Sable* is French for sandy and that describes both the texture of the final cookie and of the mixture when it is ready to shape. These cookies would keep perfectly for a few days in an airtight container – but, trust me, they will never last that long.

CHOCOLATE SABLES

MAKES 24 biscuits
PREPARATION TIME: 30 minutes, plus 2 hours chilling COOKING TIME: 12 minutes

Put the flour, cocoa powder, bicarbonate of soda and salt in a large bowl and stir to combine.

In another bowl, beat together the butter and sugars, using an electric mixer, until pale – the mixture doesn't need to be fluffy, just light and well combined. Add the flour mixture and, with the mixer on low speed, whisk together until the mixture has a sandy texture. If you mix until you have a uniform dough, the texture of the final cookie will be a bit tougher and they won't melt in the mouth. Add the chocolate and stir to combine.

Tip the mixture onto a lightly floured work surface and very gently knead to bring together to a soft dough. Divide the dough in half and roll into logs about 4cm/1½in in diameter. Wrap in cling film and chill for at least 2 hours until firm. (I normally freeze half of the dough ready to make cookies when the mood strikes.)

Preheat the oven to 180°C/350°F/Gas 4 and line two baking sheets with baking paper.

Using a thin, sharp knife, cut the log into cookies, about 1cm/½in thick. Don't worry if the cookies crumble, just press them gently back together. Put on the prepared baking sheets, slightly apart to allow them room to spread. Bake for 10–12 minutes, or until spread and lightly set around the edges but still looking undercooked in the centre.

Leave to cool on the baking sheets for 10 minutes, then transfer to a wire rack to cool completely. Store in an airtight container for up to 5 days.

275g/9¾oz/2¼ cups white spelt flour, plus extra for dusting ....
40g/1½oz/½ cup cocoa powder..........
¾ tsp bicarbonate of soda ....
1½ tsp sea salt ....
200g/7oz unsalted butter, softened .....
55g/2oz/¼ cup caster sugar ....
100g/3½oz/½ cup light soft brown sugar..
175g/6oz dark chocolate (70% cocoa solids), roughly chopped ....

Everyone loves a good carrot cake and this simple version is full of extra nutty goodness, thanks to the inclusion of wholemeal spelt flour and walnuts. The flavours perfectly complement a cup of my favourite blend of Earl Grey and lapsang souchong tea.

CARROT CAKE

MAKES 23cm/9in cake
PREPARATION TIME: 20 minutes COOKING TIME: 45 minutes

Lightly oil a 23cm/9in round cake tin and line it with baking paper. Preheat the oven to 170°C/325°F/Gas 3.

Put the eggs, sugar, vanilla, cinnamon and salt in a mixing bowl and whisk together until smooth, then add the oil, drip by drip, as if you were making a mayonnaise. Keep whisking until all the oil is added and you have a smooth emulsion. Fold in the flours and baking powder, then add the carrots, folding continuously so that you have a smooth cake batter. Add the walnuts and fold a couple of times again, then pour the mixture into the prepared cake tin.

Bake for 40–45 minutes until the cake has risen, is golden brown on top and a skewer inserted in the centre comes out clean. Transfer to a wire rack to cool.

Once the cake has cooled, make the icing. Put the cream cheese and butter in a mixing bowl and whisk together. Add the icing sugar and vanilla and whisk again until smooth. Use a spatula or palette knife to ice the carrot cake and decorate with fresh berries, fruit or nuts or other ingredients, if you like.

150ml/5fl oz/scant ⅔ cup sunflower oil, plus extra for greasing ....
3 eggs ....
150g/5½oz/heaped ¾ cup light soft brown sugar ....
1 tsp vanilla extract............................
½ tsp ground cinnamon ....
¼ tsp sea salt ....
75g/2½oz/heaped ½ cup white spelt flour ....
75g/2½oz/heaped ½ cup wholegrain spelt flour ....
1½ tsp baking powder ....
175g/6oz grated carrots ....
75g/2½oz/½ cup walnuts, coarsely chopped...

FOR THE ICING & FINISHING:
115g/4oz full-fat cream cheese............
115g/4oz unsalted butter, softened .....
115g/4oz/scant 1 cup icing sugar, sifted..
1 tsp vanilla extract............................
berries, fruit or nuts of your choice, to decorate (optional)..........................

Plums have a wonderful affinity with almonds, and this cake is so easy to rustle up that there is no excuse not to give it a go. The plums can be substituted with other seasonal stone fruit, such as greengages or apricots, if you prefer. You could also use other nuts, such as walnuts or hazelnuts, in the cake mixture, or vary the flavours by substituting the vanilla and cinnamon with freshly grated lemon or orange zest.

PLUM & FRANGIPANE CAKE

MAKES 20cm/8in cake
PREPARATION TIME: 20 minutes   COOKING TIME: 40 minutes

Preheat the oven to 180°C/350°F/Gas 4. Lightly grease a 20cm/8in round springform cake tin and dust with a little spelt flour.

Beat together the butter and sugar in a large bowl, using an electric mixer, until pale and fluffy. Add the vanilla and cinnamon and beat again. Add the eggs one at a time, including a spoonful of the flour with each egg to prevent the mixture from splitting.

Add the remaining dry ingredients to the bowl, then use a large metal spoon or spatula to fold the ingredients together so that the mixture is evenly blended. Spoon the mixture into the prepared cake tin and gently insert each plum half, cut-side down, around the cake, arranging them either in concentric circles or in whatever pattern you prefer.

Bake for 35–40 minutes until the cake is golden brown on top and a skewer inserted in the centre comes out clean. Remove from the oven and transfer to a wire rack to cool. Dust with icing sugar to serve.

150g/5½oz unsalted butter, plus extra for greasing ....
125g/5½oz/1 cup white spelt flour, plus extra for dusting ....
150g/5½oz/⅔ cup golden caster sugar
1 tsp vanilla extract.............................
¼ tsp ground cinnamon ....
3 eggs ....
125g/4½oz/1¼ cups ground almonds
1½ tsp baking powder ....
8 summer plums, such as Victoria or Opal, halved and pitted ....
a little icing sugar, sifted, for dusting ....

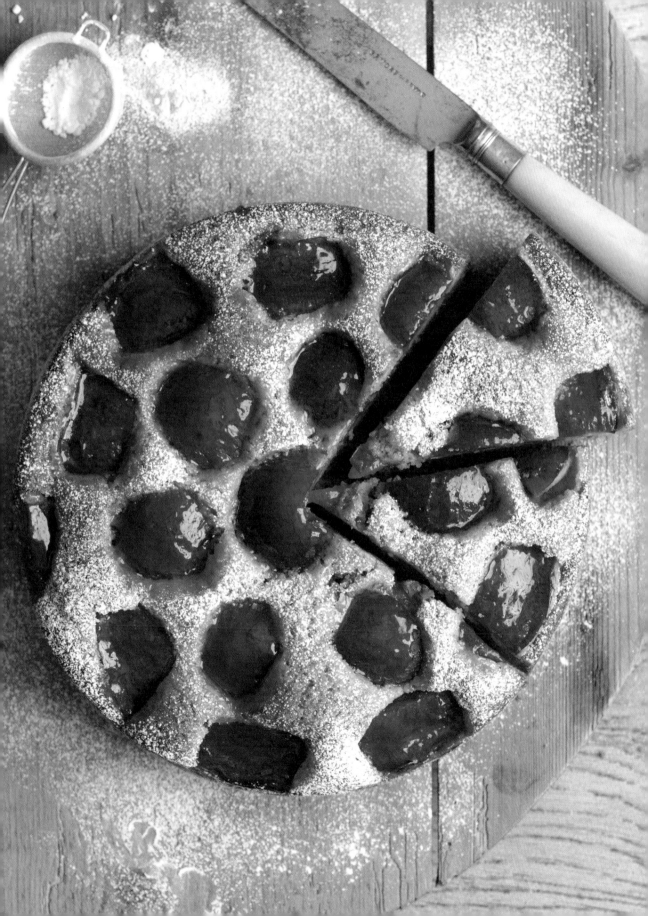

Walnuts were originally planted by the abbots of Glastonbury and have always been part of Sharpham Park's farming economy. We even found some hidden in a cavity in a stone wall in the house – with some chicken bones and clam shells – where a monk had obviously had a good lunch break 500 years ago! We planted 300 trees ten years ago to continue the tradition and now have a battle royal with the squirrels for ownership.

WALNUT & COFFEE CAKE WITH STREUSEL TOPPING

MAKES 20cm/8in sandwich cake
PREPARATION TIME: 30 minutes, plus 20 minutes cooling COOKING TIME: 1 hour

Preheat the oven to 160°C/315°F/Gas 2–3.

Put the walnuts in a roasting tin and roast for 12–14 minutes until they are light brown. Remove from the oven and leave to cool, then tip into a blender, add the oil and blitz to a dry walnut paste.

Turn the oven temperature up to 170°C/325°F/Gas 3 and line two 20cm/8in round cake tins and a baking sheet with baking paper.

Beat together the butter and sugar in a large bowl, using an electric mixer, until pale and fluffy. Add the syrup, then the eggs, one at a time, followed by the roasted walnut paste. Mix the flour, baking powder and salt in a small bowl, then fold into the mixture. Divide the cake mixture equally between the prepared cake tins.

Bake for 30 minutes, or until the top looks golden brown and feels firm to the touch. If in doubt, a skewer inserted in the centre should come out clean. Transfer to a wire rack to cool.

While the cakes are cooling, turn the oven up to 180°C/350°F/Gas 4 and scatter the topping ingredients over the prepared baking sheet. Bake for 15 minutes, or until is crisp and golden brown in colour. Remove from the oven and allow to cool before using on the top of the cake.

To make the filling and icing, beat the butter in a large bowl, using an electric mixer, until soft, then gradually add the icing sugar and beat until pale and fluffy. Add the vanilla, espresso and salt and whisk again until fluffy. Spread about one-third of the creamed mixture on top of the first sponge cake, then place the second sponge on top. Spread the remaining mix over the top and around the side of the assembled cake and scatter the toasted streusel mixture on top to serve.

FOR THE WALNUT & COFFEE CAKE:
90g/3¼oz/¾ cup walnut halves..........
3 tbsp sunflower oil...........................
215g/7½oz unsalted butter, softened
175g/6oz/scant 1 cup light soft brown sugar..
1½ tbsp golden syrup........................
3 eggs ....
220g/7¾oz/1¾ cups white spelt flour ....
2 tsp baking powder..........................
¼ tsp sea salt ....

FOR THE COFFEE FILLING & ICING:
175g/6oz unsalted butter, softened.....
250g/9oz/2 cups icing sugar, sifted.....
1 tsp vanilla extract...........................
1 espresso shot, or 3 tbsp strong coffee
¼ tsp sea salt ....

FOR THE STREUSEL TOPPING:
55g/2oz/heaped ½ cup spelt porridge flakes ....
55g/2oz unsalted butter, melted and cooled...
55g/2oz/¼ cup demerara sugar..........

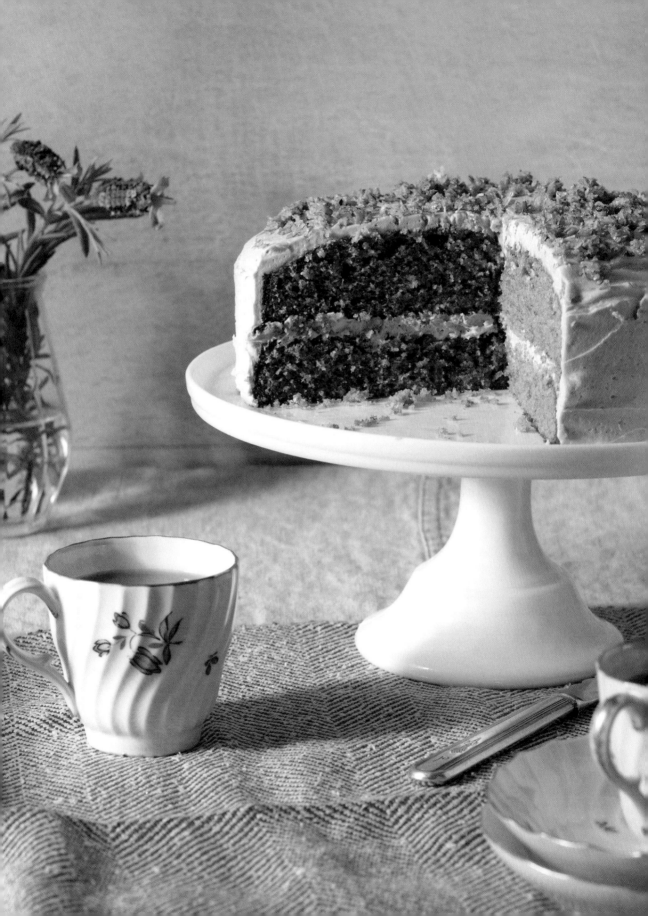

The lovely nutty taste of spelt comes through in this fabulous summer cake that features two of my favourite ingredients – raspberries and almonds. And as an added bonus, it doesn't have to be June to enjoy it, as autumn-fruiting raspberries are now widely available. You can vary this cake by using other fruits, such as blueberries or chopped rhubarb, making it perfect to adapt to whatever is in season at the time of year.

SUMMER RASPBERRY CAKE

MAKES 23cm/9in cake
PREPARATION TIME: **20 minutes** COOKING TIME: **1 hour**

Preheat the oven to 180°C/350°F/Gas 4 and grease and line a 23cm/9in round springform cake tin.

Arrange the raspberries, hole-side down, across the base of the prepared tin, wedging them in so they are tightly packed. Reserve any left over.

Beat together the butter and sugar in a large bowl, using an electric mixer, until pale and fluffy. Stir in the vanilla and the eggs, one at a time, adding a spoonful of the flour with each egg to prevent the mixture from splitting. Add the ground almonds and stir, then add the remaining flour, baking powder and salt and stir through until the mixture is evenly blended and there are no major lumps of flour. Carefully fold in any remaining raspberries, stirring once or twice.

Spoon the cake mixture into the prepared tin and smooth the top. Bake for 45–60 minutes, or until a skewer inserted in the centre comes out clean. Turn upside down onto a wire rack to cool.

Sprinkle with caster or icing sugar, if you like, and serve with double cream or crème fraîche.

175g/6oz unsalted butter, softened, plus extra for greasing ....
300g/10½oz/2 cups raspberries ....
175g/6oz/scant 1 cup light soft brown sugar ....
1 tsp vanilla extract ....
2 eggs, lightly beaten ....
200g/7oz/1⅔ cups white spelt flour....
100g/3½oz/1 cup ground almonds.....
2 tsp baking powder ....
¼ tsp sea salt ....
2 tbsp caster sugar or icing sugar, sifted, for sprinkling (optional) ....
double cream or crème fraîche, to serve ....

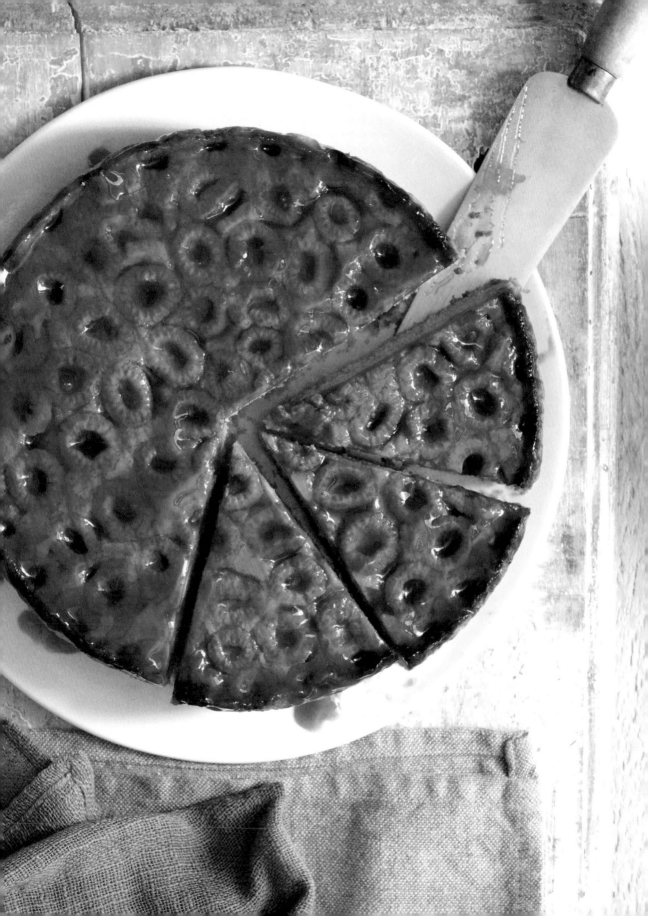

This wonderfully indulgent chocolate, rum and prune cake comes courtesy of our master-baker friend, Alex Gooch. It takes a little work in the preparation, but this moist, rich cake is very much worth the time and effort.

CHOCOLATE & RUM-SOAKED PRUNE CAKE

MAKES 20cm/8in cake
PREPARATION TIME: 30 minutes, plus 24 hours soaking and 12 hours resting COOKING TIME: 2¼ hours

Soak the prunes in the rum and 1 teaspoon of the vanilla for 24 hours.

Preheat the oven to 140°C/275°F/Gas 1. Thoroughly butter a 23cm/9in cake tin, line the base with baking paper and butter the paper. Liberally sprinkle fruit sugar on the side and base of the tin to cover the butter.

Put the chocolate in a large heatproof bowl and rest it over a saucepan of gently simmering water, making sure the bottom of the bowl does not touch the water. Heat, stirring occasionally, until the chocolate has melted.

Put the remaining butter, the ground almonds, flour, cinnamon and cocoa in a large bowl and beat together until very well mixed. Fold in the melted chocolate. In a separate bowl, whisk together the eggs and fruit sugar until pale and fluffy. Combine the mixtures and beat with a wooden spoon until it goes pale and has a creamy consistency.

Take the prunes out of the rum and squeeze to remove any excess liquid. Reserve the liquid. Chop half the prunes in half, leaving the others whole.

Put the halved prunes in the base of the prepared cake tin. Carefully spoon the cake mixture on top of the prunes, using a spatula to create an even surface. Gently push the remaining whole soaked prunes into the cake mix. Use the spatula to level the top after the whole prunes have gone in. Put the tin on a baking sheet and bake for 2¼ hours until well risen and a skewer inserted in the centre comes out clean. Leave to rest in the tin for 2 minutes, then turn the cake out upside down onto a serving plate and leave to cool for 1 hour.

Mix together the honey and the soaking rum. Pour the honey and rum mixture evenly over the top of the cake. Ideally, leave the cake to rest for at least 12 hours before serving.

350g/12oz/2 cups pitted prunes ....
150ml/5fl oz/scant ⅔ cup dark rum ...
2 tsp vanilla extract............................
190g/6¾oz unsalted butter, softened, plus extra for greasing ....
190g/6¾oz/¾ cup fruit sugar, plus extra for lining...............................
50g/1¾oz dark chocolate (70% cocoa solids), chopped...............................
110g/3¾oz/heaped 1 cup ground almonds................................
85g/3oz/⅔ cup wholegrain spelt flour ....
1 tsp ground cinnamon ....
2 tsp cocoa powder............................
3 large eggs.......................................
1 tbsp clear honey ....

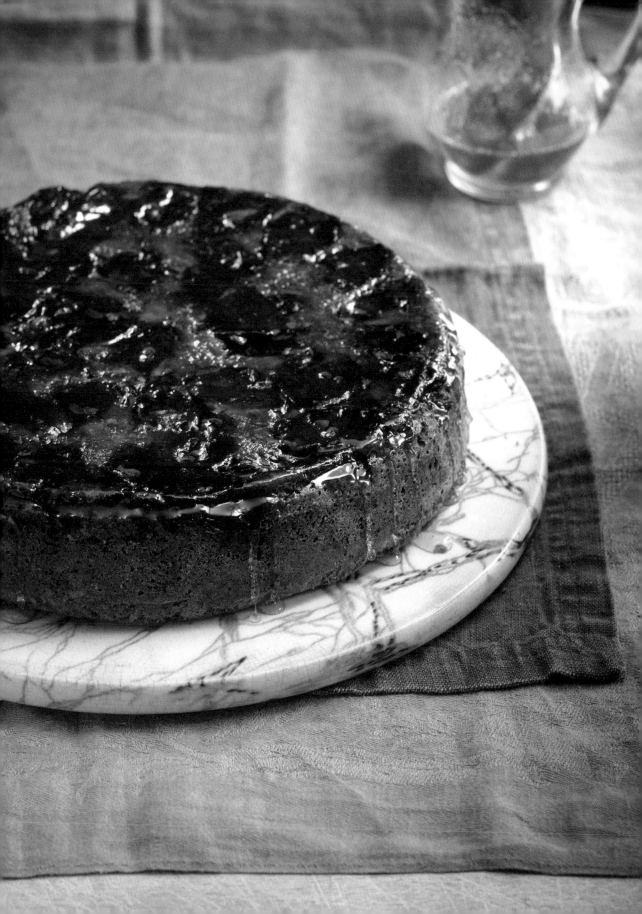

Who did first make these delicious, naughty, desirable slabs of cake? There are lots of myths, but apparently it was in the early 20th century and in Chicago, upon the request of one Bertha Palmer, who wanted a dessert smaller than a piece of cake, but easily eaten from a lunchbox! Well done, America!

DARK CHOCOLATE BROWNIE CAKE

MAKES 23cm/9in cake
PREPARATION TIME: 20 minutes COOKING TIME: 25 minutes

Preheat the oven to 180°C/350°F/Gas 4 and lightly grease and line a deep, round 23cm/9in springform cake tin with baking paper.

Put the butter in a large heatproof bowl and rest it over a saucepan of gently simmering water, making sure the bottom of the bowl does not touch the water. Add the chocolate and the salt. Heat, stirring occasionally, until the chocolate has melted. Remove from the heat and leave to one side to cool.

Meanwhile, whisk together the eggs, sugar and vanilla, using an electric mixer, until light and fluffy. Carefully pour in the chocolate mixture and the flour and fold together using figure-of-eight movements to evenly distribute all the ingredients and create a smooth batter.

Spoon the mixture into the prepared cake tin and bake for 25 minutes, or until the top of the brownie cake is crisp and separates slightly from the rest of the cake. The centre shouldn't be completely set, but beware of over-baking the cake, as it will lose its chocolate intensity the longer it stays in the oven.

Remove from the oven and transfer to a wire rack to cool.

250g/9oz unsalted butter, plus extra
  for greasing......................................
250g/9oz dark chocolate (70% cocoa
  solids), chopped.............................
½ tsp sea salt ....
7 eggs ....
250g/9oz/heaped 1 cup golden caster
  sugar..
1 tsp vanilla extract............................
125g/4½oz/1 cup white spelt flour.....

COOKS' TIP
Served warm straight from the oven, this cake also makes a delightfully rich and gooey dessert.

I am the world's greatest expert on almond slices! It's taken me years to find that perfect balance of taste and texture – and has definitely added centimetres to my waistline. With my kitchen team, Elliott and Annie at The Pantry in Kilver Court, we think we are en route to perfection – in fact, we know it!

ALMOND TART

MAKES 30 x 20cm/12 x 8in tart
PREPARATION TIME: 20 minutes, plus 10 minutes cooling COOKING TIME: 40 minutes

Preheat the oven to 150°C/300°F/Gas 2 and grease a 20 x 30cm/ 8 x 12in rectangular cake tin.

Put the flour in a large bowl, then rub in the cold butter, using your fingertips, until the mixture resembles breadcrumbs. Stir in the sugar, then the vanilla and half the honey and mix together until you have a rough dough.

Turn the dough out onto a lightly floured work surface, shape into a rectangle, then roll out so that the base fits the prepared tin. Carefully lift the pastry over the tin and use it to line the base, cutting away any excess. Prick all over with a fork.

Bake in the oven for 10 minutes, or until the base looks golden brown and feels sandy to the touch, then remove from the oven and transfer to a wire rack to cool. Once the base has cooled down, drizzle the remaining honey over the surface. Turn the oven down to 160°C/315°F/Gas 2–3

To make the topping, beat together the butter and sugar in a large bowl, using an electric mixer, until pale and fluffy. Add one egg at a time, mixing as you go, and making sure each egg is mixed in well before you add the next. Then add the almond extract, vanilla, lemon zest, flour and ground almonds, folding everything together until you have a smooth mixture.

Spread this topping over the pre-baked base and top with the flaked almonds, then bake in the oven for 25–30 minutes until the top looks golden brown, or a knife tip inserted in the centre comes out clean.

Remove from the oven and transfer to a wire rack to cool.

FOR THE BASE:
150g/5½oz cold unsalted butter, diced, plus extra for greasing............
250g/9oz/2 cups white spelt flour, plus extra for dusting ....
80g/2¾oz/⅓ cup caster sugar ....
½ tsp vanilla extract...........................
4 tbsp clear honey ....

FOR THE TOPPING:
250g/9oz unsalted butter, softened.....
250g/9oz/heaped 1 cup caster sugar ...
3 eggs ....
2 tsp almond extract...........................
1 tsp vanilla extract ....
1 tsp grated lemon zest ....
25g/1oz/2 tbsp white spelt flour ....
250g/9oz/2½ cups ground almonds ...
2 tsp flaked almonds...........................

Adam Fellows was my Michelin-starred chef at Charlton House for eight years, and one of his specialities was pâtisserrie, learnt during his career in France and Belgium. Over the years, he perfected using spelt flour in his tartlets so, for me, no spelt cookbook would be complete without one of his recipes.

MIXED BERRY TARTLETS

MAKES 4 tartlets
PREPARATION TIME: 20 minutes, plus 1 hour chilling and 10 minutes cooling COOKING TIME: 30 minutes

Put the flour in a large bowl, then rub in the cold butter, using your fingertips, until the mixture resembles fine breadcrumbs. Stir in the sugar, then the egg, then gradually add enough ice-cold water, a drop at a time, to bind everything to a smooth dough. You might need about 2 tablespoons. Cover with cling film and chill in the fridge for about 1 hour to relax the dough.

Preheat the oven to 180°C/350°F/Gas 4 and grease four 10cm/4in loose-based tartlet tins.

Turn the dough out onto a lightly floured work surface and roll out to about 5mm/¼in thick. Use to line the prepared tartlet tins and trim the edges. Line each pastry case with a piece of baking paper and cover with baking beans. Bake for 5 minutes, then remove the paper and baking beans and bake for a further 3–5 minutes until just golden. Remove the pastry cases in their tins from the oven and transfer to a wire rack to cool.

Spread the raspberry jam on the bottom of the cooled pastry cases.

To make the filling, beat together the butter and sugar in a large bowl, using an electric mixer, until pale and fluffy. Add the ground almonds and egg and mix to a smooth cream. Spoon into the pastry cases and smooth the tops. Scatter the mixed berries evenly over the top and bake for 20 minutes, or until spongy, golden and firm. Transfer to a wire rack to cool, then serve with cream or crème fraîche.

220g/7¾oz/1¾ cups white
  spelt flour ....
115g/4oz cold salted butter, diced,
  plus extra for greasing ....
1 tbsp golden caster sugar ....
1 egg, beaten ....

FOR THE RASPBERRY TOPPING:
3 tbsp raspberry or summer
  berry jam ....
100g/3½oz unsalted butter,
  softened ....
100g/3½oz/heaped ⅓ cup golden
  caster sugar ....
100g/3½oz/1 cup ground almonds.....
1 small egg ....
150g/5½oz fresh or frozen mixed
  summer berries ....
cream or crème fraîche, to serve..........

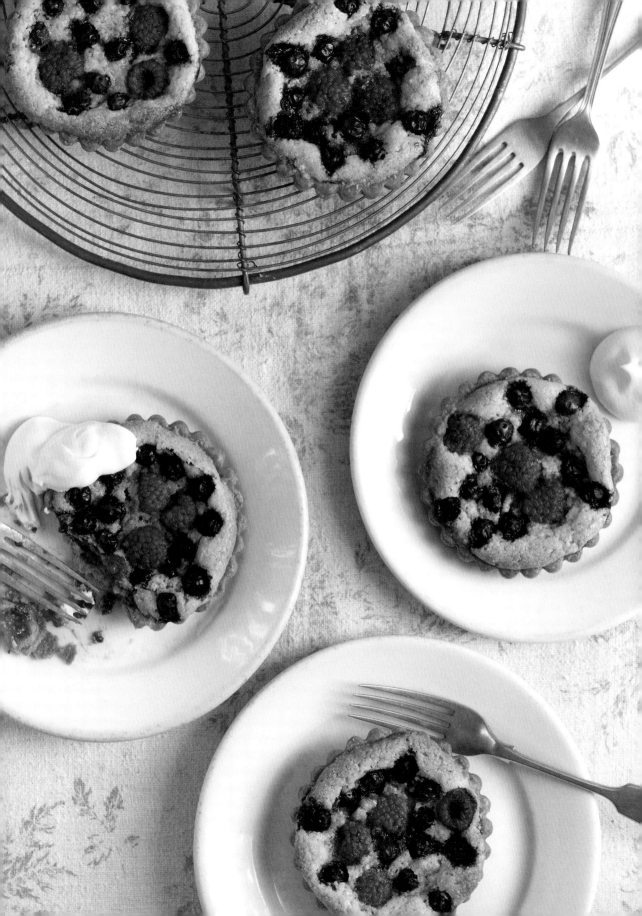

Mince pies aren't just for Christmas! As they are such a favourite in Britain, we began to experiment with making mince pies every which way very early on in our Sharpham Park spelt journey. This is our classic version, but you could well use half and half wholegrain and white flour instead of all white, or all wholegrain flour for a heavier, nuttier version.

MINCE PIES

MAKES 12 pies

PREPARATION TIME: 20 minutes, plus 1 hour chilling COOKING TIME: 15 minutes

Put the flour in a large bowl, then rub in the cold butter, using your fingertips, until the mixture resembles fine breadcrumbs. Stir in the caster sugar, then the egg, then gradually add enough ice-cold water, a drop at a time, to bind everything to a smooth dough. Cover with cling film and chill for about 1 hour to relax the dough.

Preheat the oven to 180°C/350°F/Gas 4 and lightly grease a 12-hole cupcake tin.

Turn the dough out onto a lightly floured work surface and roll out to 5mm/¼in thick. Cut out shapes with an 8cm/3¼in cutter and use to line the holes of the pan. Spoon in the mince pie filling. Cut little strips of leftover dough and criss-cross them on top of the mince filling, moistening the edges to stick them to the pastry bases.

Bake the pies for 10–15 minutes until the pastry is sandy to the touch and golden in colour. Transfer to a wire rack to cool, then dust with icing sugar to serve.

220g/7¾oz/1¾ cups white spelt flour ....
115g/4oz cold unsalted butter, plus extra for greasing ....
1 tbsp golden caster sugar...................
1 egg, beaten ....
450g/1lb mince pie filling ....
icing sugar, sifted, for dusting............

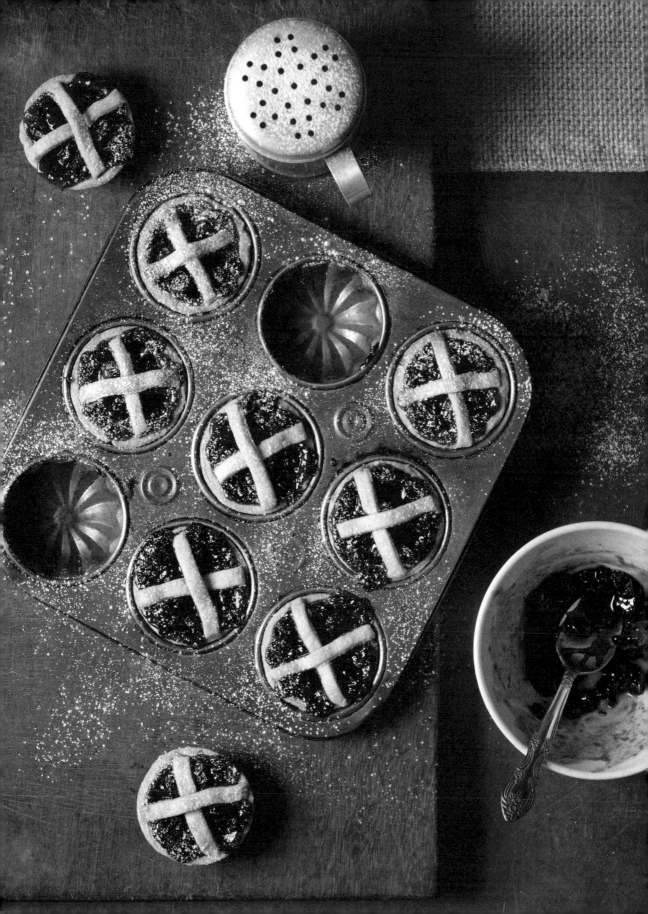

Your patience will be rewarded if you have taken the time to chill this traybake thoroughly for a few hours in the fridge before slicing it into squares, as it will set much better. Either way, the texture has a delicious, delicate crunch that is perfect with a cup of strong coffee.

MAPLE & PECAN SQUARES

MAKES 9 squares
PREPARATION TIME: 15 minutes, plus 2 hours chilling COOKING TIME: 30 minutes

Preheat the oven to 180°C/350°F/Gas 4 and line a 23cm/9in square cake tin with baking paper.

Put the butter, sugar, maple syrup, vanilla, cinnamon and salt in a saucepan over a low heat and bring slowly to a simmer, allowing everything to melt and mix together. Add the pecans and the spelt porridge flakes and stir well.

Spoon the mixture into the prepared cake tin, smooth the top so that it is as even as possible, and bake for 30 minutes, or until the top looks golden brown and slightly crisp.

Leave to cool in the tin. Once cool, put the traybake, still in the tin, in the fridge for a few hours or overnight to set fully before slicing into squares. These will keep in an airtight tin at room temperature for about a week (if they last that long).

150g/5½oz unsalted butter.................
125g/4½oz/⅔ cup light muscovado sugar...
115g/4oz/⅓ cup maple syrup.............
1 tsp vanilla extract...........................
½ tsp ground cinnamon.....................
¼ tsp sea salt ....
150g/5½oz/1½ cups pecans ....
150g/5½oz/1½ cups spelt porridge flakes ....

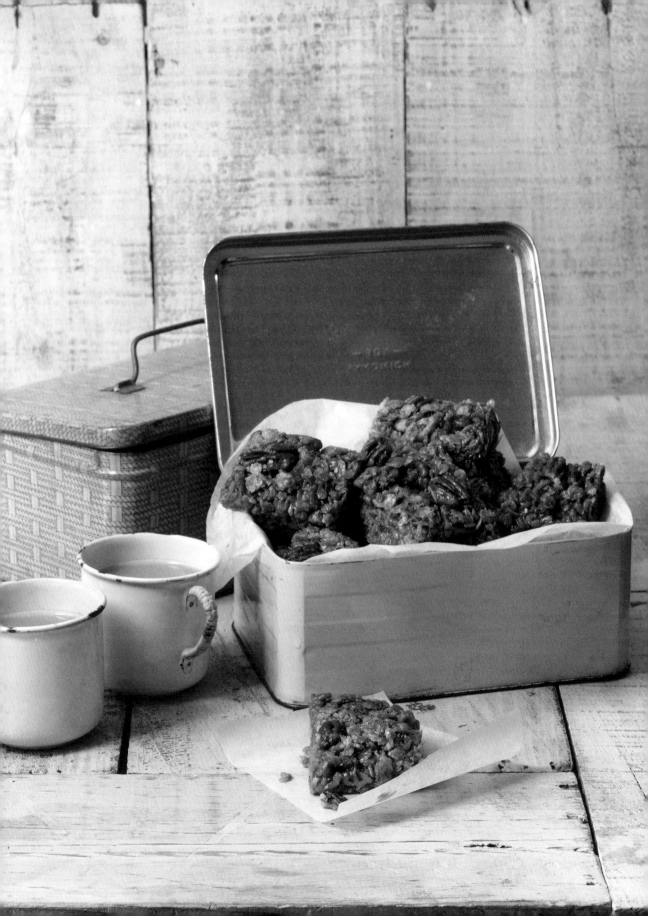

A first-of-the-season fruit, rhubarb has a lovely sharp flavour. We grow it in the old-fashioned way, under terracotta cloches, which forces the stalks, making them slender, sweeter and more tender.

RHUBARB TRAYBAKE

MAKES 30 x 20cm/12 x 8in traybake
PREPARATION TIME: 15 minutes COOKING TIME: 50 minutes

Preheat the oven to 180°C/350°F/Gas 4 and lightly butter a 25 x 20cm/12 x 8in rectangular cake tin.

Put the rhubarb in a large saucepan and sprinkle with 2 tablespoons of the sugar and the orange juice, reserving the zest for the cake mixture. Bring to the boil, then turn the heat down to low and simmer gently for 5 minutes. Leave to one side.

Beat together the butter and remaining sugar in a large bowl, using an electric mixer, until pale and fluffy. Add the eggs one at a time, including a spoonful of the flour with each egg to prevent the mixture from splitting. Add the remaining flours with the ground almonds, baking powder, bicarbonate of soda, spices, salt and orange zest and blend together. Stir in the soured cream, using a large metal spoon, making a figure-of-eight motion in the mixture until it is fully combined. Spoon the mixture into the prepared cake tin and top with the rhubarb.

Bake in the centre of the oven for 35–45 minutes, or until the traybake is golden brown and firm to the touch. A skewer inserted in the centre should come out clean. Transfer to a wire rack to cool. Cut into squares and serve with a spoonful of soured cream, if you like.

175g/6oz unsalted butter, softened, plus extra for greasing ....

6 sticks of rhubarb, chopped into 2.5cm/1in chunks...........................

270g/9½oz/scant 1¼ cups golden caster sugar ....

grated zest and juice of 1 orange........

3 eggs ....

175g/6oz/1⅓ cups white spelt flour....

75g/2½oz/heaped ½ cup wholegrain spelt flour ....

75g/2½oz/¾ cup ground almonds .....

2 tsp baking powder ....

¼ tsp bicarbonate of soda.................

1 tsp ground cinnamon ....

1 tsp vanilla extract...........................

¼ tsp salt..

150ml/5fl oz/scant ⅔ cup soured cream or Greek yogurt, plus extra for serving (optional) ....

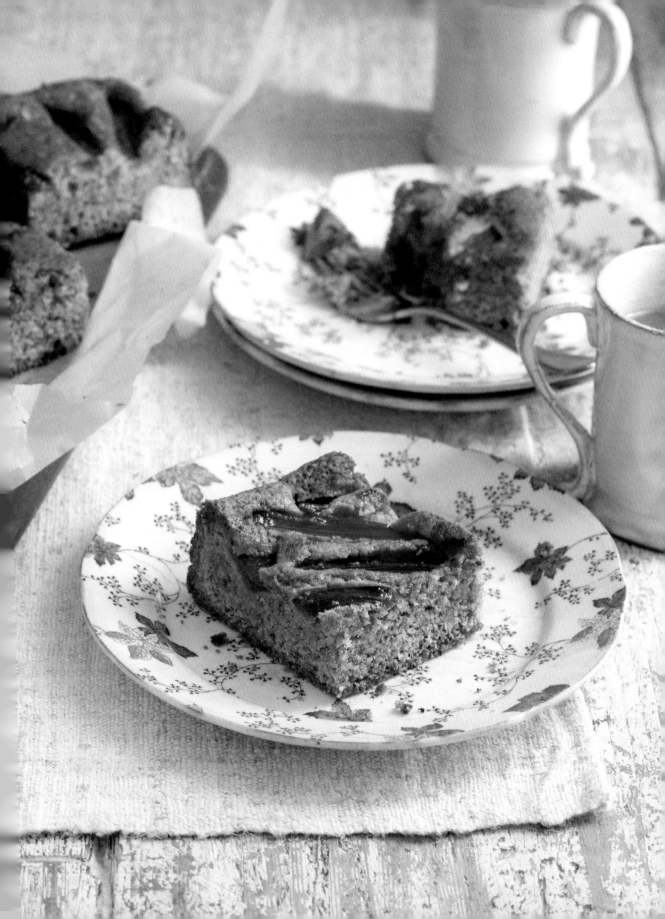

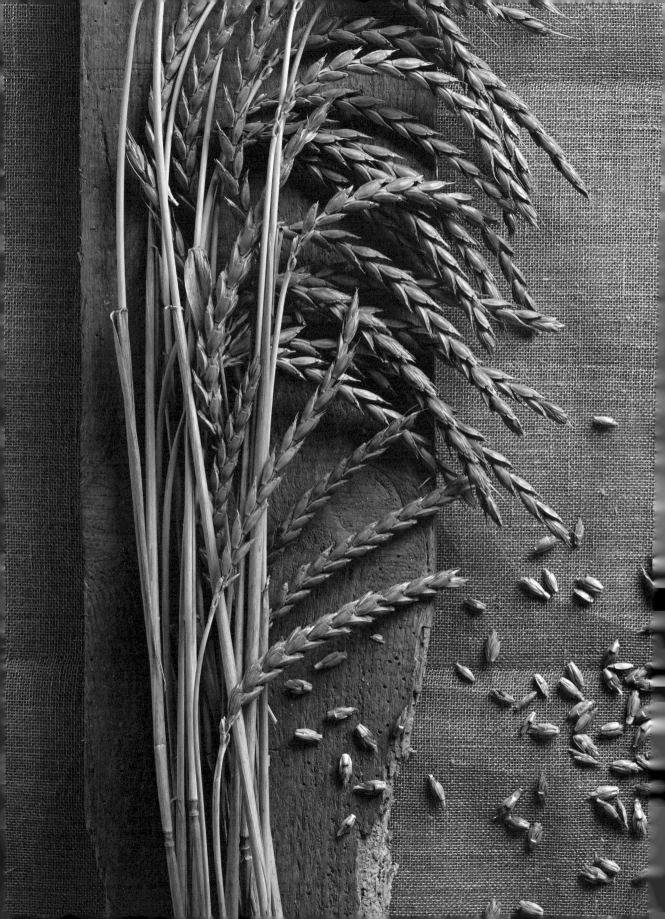

MAIN MEALS

Once again, pearled spelt is very much the hero of this chapter. Wonderfully absorbent, it soaks up the juices of anything you pair it with, whether it is Lamb Shanks with Pearled Spelt (see page 128), Lemon & Almond Cod with Spelt & Asparagus (see page 143) or Speltotto (see page 136), a wonderful invention where the grain takes on the creamy consistency of risotto rice.

There are other Italian-inspired favourites too, such as Gnocchi with Walnut & Basil Pesto (see page 144), and Pork & Fennel Meatballs in Tomato Sauce with Spaghetti (see page 131). But there's nothing to beat a good home-grown traditional English recipe, and what can come closer to Sharpham Park than Venison Wellington (see page 134)? I like to imagine the red deer grazing the forests and fields in the thirteenth century, brought to the table after an energetic day's hunting. In this recipe you can use either a whole fillet or tenderloin of venison – either way it's the healthiest of meats. Wrap it in a spelt pancake, roll it in puff pastry, and you have a feast fit for a king, or should I say an abbot?

The only time I was ever lampooned in *Private Eye* magazine (thank goodness!) was with a quote taken from our then current Mulberry Home brochure: 'To the British, the dining room is far more than a mere accessory to the kitchen, it is a theatre of extravagance!' I'd like to think that the British have got better and better at creating great food, not just great theatre. And spelt certainly deserves star billing.

Sven-Hanson Britt, another great Scandinavian chef, gave me this recipe. Why are there so many good Scandinavian chefs – or is it that I am drawn to their cooking style! It has a lovely golden topping and a rich, flavoursome filling.

CHICKEN, LEEK & KALE PIE

SERVES 4
PREPARATION TIME: 40 minutes, plus making the pastry COOKING TIME: 30 minutes

Roll out the rested pastry on a lightly floured surface into a sheet or circle to fit the top of a deep oval pie dish with a rim. Keep the trimmings for other pastry items or for pie decorations.

To make the filling, put the thigh meat and prunes in a food processor with 1 teaspoon of the mustard, the salt and pepper. Pulse until chopped enough to form into small balls, shape them and set aside. Preheat the oven to 180°C/350°F/Gas 4.

Melt the butter in a large saucepan over a low heat. Add the flour and cook for about a minute, then slowly whisk in the stock. Add the remaining mustard and the chopped parsley, then season to taste with salt and pepper. A splash of sherry is also a good addition. Add the leeks to the sauce and simmer for a few minutes until starting to soften. The sauce should be reasonably thick but not gloopy. Add the kale and stir again.

Add the chunks of chicken breast and the thigh dumplings to the sauce and put into an ovenproof dish to which a pastry lid can be easily attached. Lay the rolled pastry on top and decorate with pastry trimmings if you feel the need or have the time. Brush with a little milk to glaze, if you like.

Bake for 30 minutes, or until the pastry is flaky and looks golden brown. Remove from the oven and allow to cool slightly before serving.

1 recipe quantity Rough Puff Pastry
  (see page 15).....................................
a little white spelt flour, for dusting....

FOR THE FILLING:
2 chicken thighs, skinned
  and boned ....
4 prunes, pitted, preferably Agen........
2 tsp Dijon mustard ....
55g/2oz unsalted butter.....................
60g/2¼oz/½ cup white spelt flour......
500ml/17fl oz/2 cups chicken stock ...
2 tbsp chopped parsley ....
a splash of dry sherry, such as fino or
  manzanilla (optional)......................
2 large leeks, trimmed and cut into
  1cm/½in thick slices ....
2 large kale sprigs, spines removed,
  finely chopped ....
2 skinless, boneless chicken breasts,
  cut into chunks...............................
a little milk or beaten egg, to glaze
  (optional) ....
sea salt and freshly ground black
  pepper ....

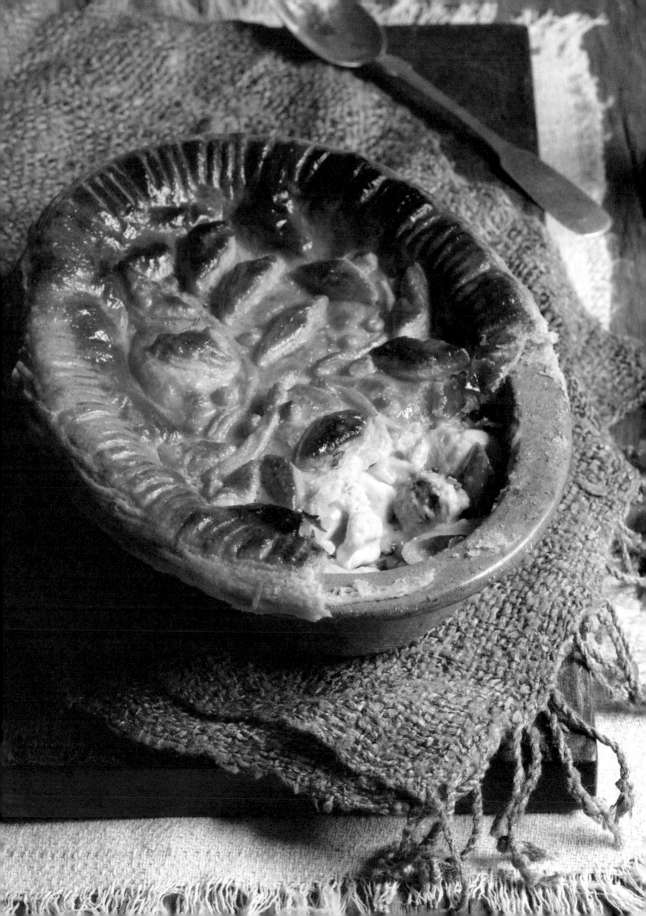

Try to buy free-range or organic chicken if you can, so there are no pesticides on the grain they eat. Pearled spelt is so versatile and makes a fabulous base for stuffing the bird, taking up all the delicious flavours from the meat.

ROAST CHICKEN WITH PEARLED SPELT STUFFING

SERVES 4

PREPARATION TIME: 35 minutes COOKING TIME: 2½ hours

Cook the pearled spelt in boiling water for 20 minutes, or until tender, following the packet instructions. Drain and leave to cool slightly.

To make the stuffing, melt the butter in a large pan over a medium heat, add the onions and garlic and fry for 5 minutes until transparent. Scrape the thyme leaves off their twigs, add them to the mixture and cook for a further 2 minutes. Add the cooked spelt and the grated chestnuts. Take the pan off the heat and add the chopped parsley. Fold in the egg and the breadcrumbs and season the mixture generously with salt and pepper. Leave to one side to cool.

Preheat the oven to 200°C/400°F/Gas 6.

Put all the stuffing into the cavity of the chicken and truss the legs together using kitchen string so that you seal in the spelt stuffing. Put thin strips of butter underneath the chicken skin, especially around the breast meat, which tends to dry out, then season the whole bird with salt and pepper.

Put the chicken in a roasting tin and roast for 30 minutes until the skin is starting to brown, then turn the oven down to 180°C/350°F/Gas 4 and roast for a further 15 minutes.

In a large bowl, toss the vegetables in the oil and season with salt and pepper. Scatter them into the roasting tin, around and under the chicken, then roast for a further 1–1¼ hours until the chicken is cooked through and the juices run clear when the thickest part of the thigh is pierced with the tip of a sharp knife.

Lift the chicken out of the tin onto a serving plate, cover with kitchen foil and leave to rest in a warm place. Turn the oven down to 140°C/275°F/Gas 1 to keep the vegetables warm until you are ready to carve and serve the chicken.

1.5kg–2kg/3lb 5oz–4lb 8oz chicken ...
50g/1¾oz unsalted butter ....
assorted vegetables, such as onions, carrots, sweet potatoes, parsnips, swede, cauliflower, turnips, peeled and cut into chunks or batons ....
3 tbsp olive oil ....
sea salt and freshly ground black pepper ....

FOR THE STUFFING:
150g/5½oz/heaped ¾ cup pearled spelt ....
150g/5½oz unsalted butter, softened ..
200g/7oz onions, finely chopped ....
2 garlic cloves, finely chopped ....
3 large thyme sprigs ....
100g/3½oz cooked peeled chestnuts, grated ....
1 small handful of chopped parsley .....
2 eggs, lightly beaten ....
50g/1¾oz/1 cup fresh spelt breadcrumbs ....

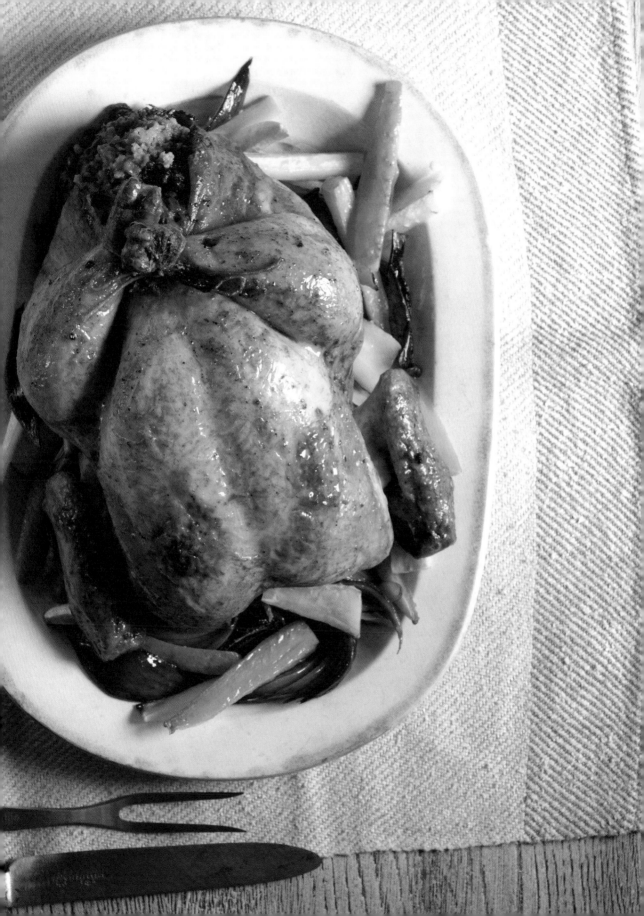

Right from the start, we wanted to have the best-tasting meat to serve farm-to-fork dishes in our restaurant so, having consulted with the best local butchers, we settled on Hebridean and Manx Loughtan sheep. Though small, the animals mature with a really good marbling to the meat, especially when fed a diet with extra spelt bran from our mill. This dish is one of my favourites.

LAMB SHANKS WITH PEARLED SPELT

SERVES 4

PREPARATION TIME: 20 minutes   COOKING TIME: 3½ hours

Preheat the oven to 140°C/275°F/Gas 1.

Season the flour generously with salt and pepper. Roll the lamb shanks in the seasoned flour until coated. Heat the oil in a heavy-based frying pan over a medium heat, add the lamb and fry until the meat is coloured all over.

Transfer the lamb to a deep roasting dish and add the chopped vegetables, garlic, rosemary and anchovies. Blend the tomato purée with the wine and Worcestershire sauce and add it to the pan, then add just enough stock to cover the lamb and vegetables. Cover the dish loosely with kitchen foil and cook in the oven for 3 hours. The lamb shanks should be soft and the meat should come off the bone easily.

Meanwhile, cook the pearled spelt in boiling water for 20 minutes, or until tender, following the packet instructions. Drain.

Lift the lamb out of the dish, cover with kitchen foil and leave to one side. Strain the cooking liquid through a fine sieve into a saucepan and discard the vegetables. Bring the sauce to the boil over a high heat and boil for a few minutes until reduced by about half. Stir in the honey for extra stickiness and the butter for gloss, too, if you like.

Turn the heat down to low, add the cooked pearled spelt to the sauce and warm through, then add the lamb shanks, cover them with the sauce and gently warm through before serving with seasonal vegetables of your choice, such as carrots, broccoli or peas, or a fresh green salad with herbs.

4 lamb shanks ....
125g/4½oz/1 cup white spelt flour.....
2 tbsp olive oil....................................
10 tomatoes, roughly chopped ....
1 head of celery, roughly chopped ......
3 onions, roughly chopped ....
1 leek, trimmed and roughly chopped .
3 large carrots, roughly chopped.........
1 garlic clove, crushed ....
1 large rosemary sprig........................
50g/1¾oz/½ small jar Spanish or
    Italian anchovies, drained and
    chopped..
1 tsp tomato purée ....
600ml/21fl oz/scant 2½ cups red
    wine..
1 tbsp Worcestershire sauce ....
about 500ml/17fl oz/2 cups lamb or
    vegetable stock or water ....
200g/7oz/heaped 1 cup pearled spelt..
1 tbsp clear honey ....
1 tbsp unsalted butter (optional) ....
sea salt and freshly ground black
    pepper ....
seasonal vegetables or fresh green
    salad herbs, to serve ....

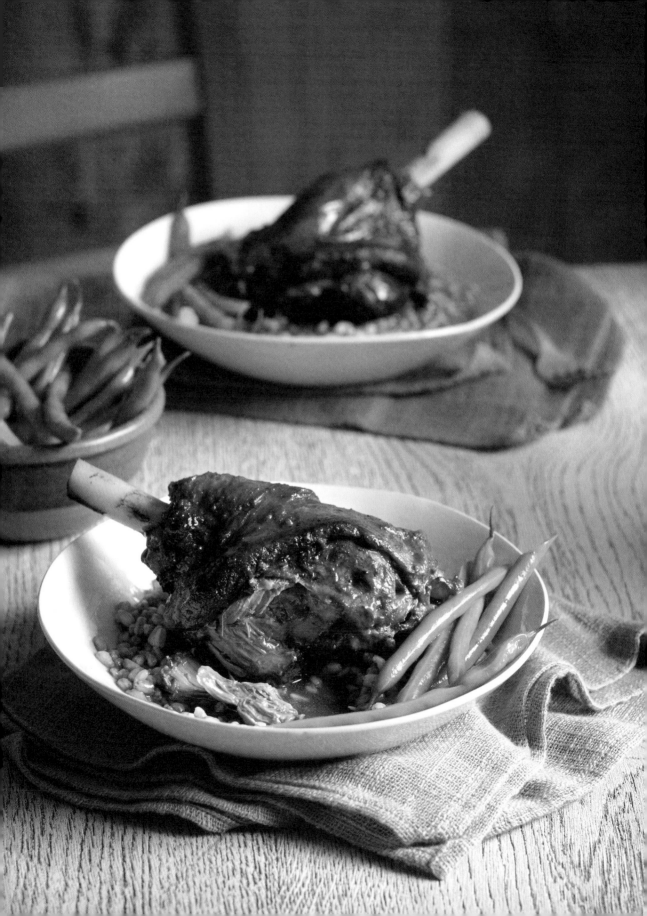

This is a real showstopper of a dish, ideally served during the winter months on account of its rich, warming spices, but, to be honest, it can be eaten any time of the year. Ask your butcher for beef cheeks – I think they are underrated – but if you can't get them, use brisket or any cut suitable for braising.

SPICED BEEF HOTPOT

SERVES 4
PREPARATION TIME: 20 minutes COOKING TIME: 3½ hours

Preheat the oven to 150°C/300°F/Gas 2.

Season the flour generously with salt and pepper. Roll the beef in the seasoned flour until coated. Heat the oil in a heavy-based frying pan over a medium heat, add the beef and fry until the meat is coloured all over. Do this in batches.

Transfer the beef to a deep roasting dish and add the harissa, chopped vegetables, garlic and herbs. Blend the tomato purée with the porter, Worcestershire sauce, treacle and mustard and add it to the pan, then add just enough stock to cover the beef and vegetables. Cover the dish loosely with kitchen foil and cook in the oven for 3 hours. The beef cheeks will be tender and the sauce a deep, dark colour.

Meanwhile, cook the pearled spelt in boiling water for 20 minutes, or until tender, following the packet instructions. Drain.

Lift the beef and vegetables out of the sauce and leave to one side. Discard the thyme sprig and bay leaves. Bring the sauce to the boil over a high heat and cook until reduced by about half.

Turn the heat down to low, add the cooked pearled spelt to the sauce and warm through, then return the beef and vegetables to the pan and gently warm through before serving with a fresh seasonal salad of your favourite ingredients.

125g/4½oz/1 cup white spelt flour.....
2 beef cheeks, about 450g/1lb each, or brisket or braising steak, cut into chunks..
2 tbsp olive oil....................................
2 tbsp harissa paste ....
400g/14oz/1⅔ cups tinned chopped tomatoes..
1 head of fennel, trimmed and roughly chopped............................
2 red onions, roughly chopped..........
1 red pepper, deseeded and sliced ....
1 green pepper, deseeded and sliced....
2 garlic cloves, crushed ....
1 bunch of thyme.............................
2 bay leaves ....
1 tsp tomato purée ....
600ml/21fl oz/scant 2½ cups porter, or similar dark beer........................
1 tbsp Worcestershire sauce ....
1 tbsp black treacle...........................
1 tbsp coarsegrain mustard ....
300ml/10½fl oz/scant 1¼ cups beef or vegetable stock or water..............
200g/7oz/heaped 1 cup pearled spelt..
sea salt and freshly ground black pepper ....
a fresh green salad, to serve...............

The title of this recipe has memories of school meals and rubber meatballs that you could bounce off the wall (and we did!), but nothing could be further from the truth. Despite what you may have experienced at school, this has to be one of the best basic recipes.

PORK & FENNEL MEATBALLS IN TOMATO SAUCE WITH SPAGHETTI

SERVES 4
PREPARATION TIME: 20 minutes, plus making the pasta COOKING TIME: 45 minutes

Make and roll out the pasta (see page 16), then put it through a pasta machine to make the spaghetti. Put the pork mince in a large bowl. Soak the breadcrumbs in the milk and yogurt in a small bowl while you prepare the remaining ingredients.

Heat the sunflower oil in a frying pan over a medium-low heat, add the shallots and chilli and fry for 5 minutes, or until soft. Add the garlic and cook for 1 minute, then stir in the fennel seeds. Cook over a low heat for 1 minute, then remove from the pan and leave to cool slightly. Stir it into the pork mince and add the soaked breadcrumbs. Season with salt and pepper and bring the mixture together until blended.

To test the seasoning, shape a spoonful of the mixture into a 2cm/¾in meatball and fry in a little oil for a few minutes until browned. Taste the meatball and adjust the seasoning of the remaining mixture, if you like. Shape the remaining mixture into bite-sized meatballs.

Heat the olive oil for the meatballs in a large frying pan and fry the meatballs for 10 minutes, turning, or until cooked and golden.

Meanwhile, heat the sunflower oil in a saucepan over a medium heat and fry the onion for 6 minutes, or until soft. Add the garlic and fry for 1 minute, then stir in the tomatoes and passata and cook for 20 minutes, or until reduced by half. Season with salt and pepper, add the basil and chilli flakes, if using, and cook for 5 minutes. Remove from the heat, stir in a little olive oil to give a glossy texture and add the meatballs. Cover and leave to one side while you cook the spaghetti.

Bring a large saucepan of lightly salted water to the boil. Add the spelt spaghetti and cook for 3 minutes for fresh or 7 minutes for dried pasta, or until al dente, then drain. Serve the meatballs and sauce on a bed of pasta, sprinkled with Parmesan and drizzled with olive oil.

½ recipe quantity Pasta (see page 16) or shop-bought spelt pasta ....
500g/1lb 2oz pork mince ....
50g/1¾oz/1 cup fresh spelt breadcrumbs........................
3 tbsp full-fat milk ....
1 tbsp natural yogurt ....
1 tbsp sunflower oil, plus extra for testing.............................
1 banana shallot, finely chopped.........
1 large green chilli, deseeded and finely chopped ....
1 garlic clove, finely chopped.............
2 tbsp fennel seeds.........................
1 tbsp olive oil, plus extra to serve ......
freshly grated Parmesan cheese, for sprinkling ....
sea salt and freshly ground black pepper ....

FOR THE TOMATO SAUCE:
1 tbsp sunflower oil ....
1 large Spanish onion, chopped.........
2 garlic cloves, finely chopped ....
500g/1lb 2oz plum tomatoes, skinned and chopped.....................
500g/1lb 2oz passata ....
1 bunch of basil leaves......................
a pinch of chilli flakes (optional) ....
a drizzle of olive oil..........................

Fajita was originally a Mexican meat cut, probably skirt (which can be very good) but has now morphed into being a Texan/Mexican restaurant dish. Our fajitas are made with pork, wrapped in spelt tortillas, although you could substitute them with chapatis, depending where you are in the world. Whatever you choose to call them, they are always a reliable and excellent dish.

MEXICAN PORK FAJITAS

SERVES 4
PREPARATION TIME: 15 minutes, plus 1 hour marinating COOKING TIME: 20 minutes

To make the marinade, put the lime zest and juice, sugar, spices and a generous seasoning of salt and pepper into a non-metallic bowl and stir together. Add the pork and rub the marinade into all the pork slices. Cover with cling film and chill in the fridge for 1 hour.

When you're ready to start cooking the fajita filling, preheat the oven to its lowest setting. Cover the spelt wraps in kitchen foil and place them in the warm oven.

Put 2 tablespoons of the oil in a large frying pan or wok and cook the onions and peppers over a medium heat for 10 minutes, or until soft. Remove the vegetables and keep them warm in the oven. Drain any excess marinade from the pork slices. Add another tablespoon of oil to the same pan and turn the heat up to high. Cook the pork in batches for 2–3 minutes to sear the outside of the meat. Remove from the pan and repeat with the remaining batches.

Keep the pork warm in the oven, while you peel, pit and slice the avocados, roughly chop the coriander and quarter the limes.

Serve the warm spelt wraps on individual plates and let everyone help themselves to the first round of filling, garnishing with avocado, coriander, a squeeze of lime juice and a spoonful of soured cream before rolling up and eating.

1 pork tenderloin, thinly sliced...........
1 recipe quantity Spelt Wraps (see page 81), made into 8 small wraps...
4 tbsp sunflower oil ....
2 Spanish onions, thinly sliced ....
1 green pepper, deseeded and thinly sliced ....
1 red pepper, deseeded and thinly sliced ....
1 yellow pepper, deseeded and thinly sliced ....
2 ripe avocados.................................
1 bunch of coriander leaves ....
4 limes ....
300ml/10½fl oz/scant 1¼ cups soured cream ....
sea salt and freshly ground black pepper ....

FOR THE LIME MARINADE:
grated zest and juice of 1 lime ....
2 garlic cloves, finely crushed.............
1 tbsp light soft brown sugar ....
1 tsp ground cumin...........................
1 tsp paprika ....
½ tsp cayenne...................................

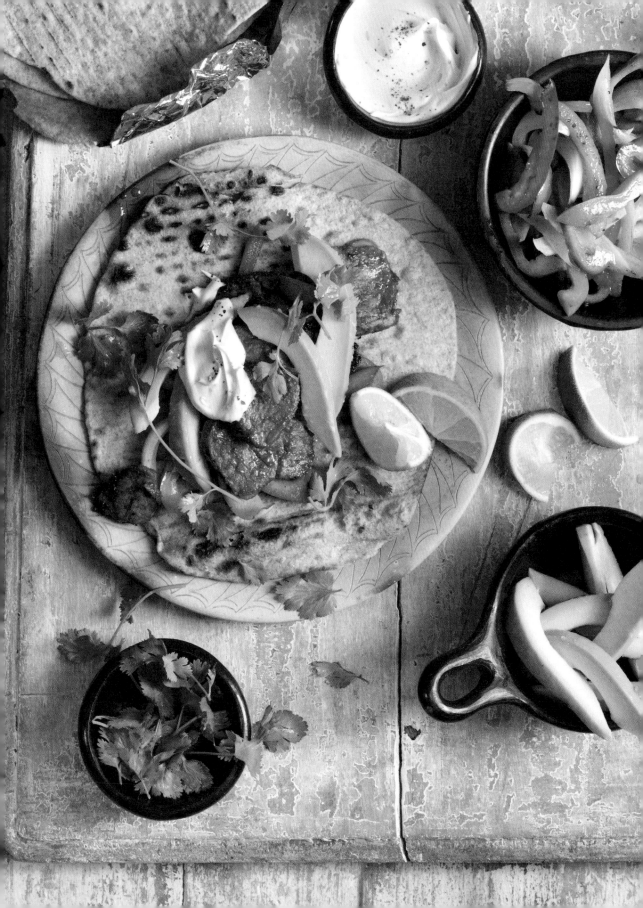

Always a crowd-pleaser, this venison Wellington makes an impressive dish to serve to guests. The lean tenderloin is also very good for you – a fact long recognized at Sharpham Park. The first red deer were introduced to the land in the 12th century, when the abbots of Glastonbury would invite their guests to hunt and then enjoy a major feast.

VENISON WELLINGTON

SERVES 4–6
PREPARATION TIME: 1 hour, plus 20 minutes resting COOKING TIME: 1 hour

To make the pancakes, put the flour, salt and sugar in a large bowl and make a well in the centre. Add the eggs and half the milk and beat, using an electric mixer, until really smooth. Add the remaining milk and whisk to a smooth batter.

To make the filling, heat the oil in a frying pan, add the shallots and fry gently for 5 minutes, or until soft. Add the mushrooms and cook until all the excess liquid has evaporated. Season with salt and pepper to taste.

Melt a knob of butter in a 25cm/10in frying pan until sizzling. Add about one-third of the batter to cover the pan about 3mm/⅛in deep and cook until bubbling. Flip the pancake and cook the other side for 30 seconds, then remove it from the pan and leave to cool. Make 2 more pancakes in the same way.

Weigh the meat and calculate the cooking time. Heat a large frying pan over a high heat, then sear the whole fillet very quickly to keep all the meat juices inside. Remove from the heat and leave to cool. Preheat the oven to 170°C/325°F/Gas 3 and grease a large baking sheet.

Put your pancakes overlapping on a work surface so that they are long enough to cover the entire fillet. Spread with the mushroom mixture. Put the fillet on top and completely wrap the fillet in the pancakes.

Roll the pastry out thinly on a lightly floured work surface, then wrap the fillet and pancakes completely in a sheet of puff pastry, brushing the edges with a little egg to seal the parcel. Brush a thin layer of egg over the pastry, then wrap it in the second sheet of pastry, sealing the ends with egg wash. Ensure that there are no air bubbles, as the pastry must be completely smooth. Brush with the remaining egg wash.

Put the parcel on the prepared baking sheet and roast at 15 minutes per 450g/1lb. Leave to rest for 20 minutes in a warm place. Slice into 3cm/1¼in slices and serve immediately with seasonal vegetables.

25g/1oz butter, plus extra for greasing
1 whole fillet or tenderloin of venison, about 1kg/2lb 4oz in weight ....
1 recipe quantity Rough Puff Pastry (see page 15) or 425g/15oz packet of ready-rolled puff pastry sheets......
a little white spelt flour, for dusting ....
1 egg, beaten ....
seasonal vegetables, to serve ....

FOR THE PANCAKES:
150g/5½oz/scant 1¼ cups white spelt flour ....
a pinch of sea salt ....
1 tbsp caster sugar ....
2 eggs ....
350ml/12fl oz/scant 1½ cups full-fat milk ....

FOR THE FILLING:
1 tbsp olive oil...................................
2 shallots, chopped............................
500g/1lb 2oz wild mushrooms ....
sea salt and freshly ground black pepper ....

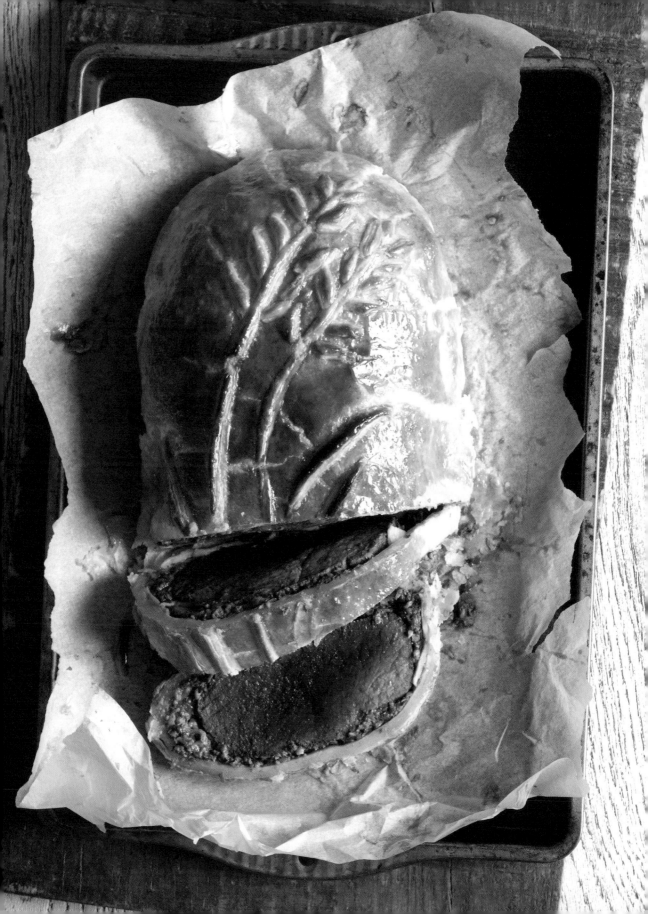

Pearled spelt makes the most delicious, creamy dishes similar to a risotto – hence the fact that we call them 'speltotto'. The great benefit of pearled spelt over rice is that it more readily absorbs flavours, so you can use it to bring alive any leftovers from the weekend roast. We've given you three versions to start, but do experiment yourself with any ingredients you might have, switching in meat, fish or whatever vegetables are in season.

SPELTOTTO

SERVES 4
PREPARATION TIME: **10 minutes** COOKING TIME: about 25 minutes
(depending on the variation)

Start by making the speltotto base. Heat the oil in a large frying pan over a medium heat. Add the shallots and fry for about 3 minutes until soft and translucent. Add the pearled spelt and gently sauté for 2 minutes, stirring constantly so the spelt is coated in the hot oil and doesn't stick to the pan. Add the wine and continue to stir.

Reduce the heat to a low simmer. Begin to add the chicken stock a little at a time, adding just enough to cover the pearled spelt, then waiting for it to absorb the liquid before adding more. Continue in this way for about 7 minutes until almost all the stock listed for the base has been absorbed.

From this point, continue with one of the variations.

2 tbsp olive oil.....................................
3 shallots, finely chopped ....
200g/7oz/heaped 1 cup pearled
    spelt..
200ml/7fl oz/scant 1 cup dry white or
    red wine...
500ml/17fl oz/2 cups hot chicken or
    vegetable stock...............................

GREEN SPELTOTTO

Continue to simmer the speltotto base in the pan, and add the additional hot stock as you did for the speltotto base, waiting for a spoonful to be absorbed before adding more, until all the stock has been absorbed. Simmer for a few more minutes, if necessary, until the pearled spelt is tender.

Add half the butter and the walnut pesto and stir through. Season to taste with salt and pepper and stir the blanched broccoli into the speltotto. Add the Parmesan and the remaining butter, stirring so that all the ingredients are evenly distributed. Serve hot.

500ml/17fl oz/2 cups hot chicken or
    vegetable stock...............................
50g/2oz unsalted butter, plus extra
    for finishing.....................................
4 tbsp Walnut & Basil Pesto
    (see page 144)................................
1 head of broccoli, chopped into
    florets and blanched........................
60g/2¼oz/⅔ cup freshly grated
    Parmesan ....
sea salt and freshly ground black
    pepper ....

WILD MUSHROOM & ROAST CHICKEN SPELTOTTO

Continue to simmer the speltotto base in the pan, and add the additional hot stock as you did for the speltotto base, waiting for a spoonful to be absorbed before adding more, until all the stock has been absorbed. Simmer for a few more minutes, if necessary, until the pearled spelt is tender.

Meanwhile, melt 50g/1¾oz of the butter with a little olive oil in a saucepan with the thyme sprigs and garlic. Once the butter is foaming, remove the thyme sprigs and the garlic so that they don't burn, then add the wild mushrooms, season with salt and pepper and cook over a medium heat for 5 minutes until most of the liquid has evaporated and they caramelize slightly. Add the chicken and stir until heated through, then add the crème fraîche and stir until the mixture thickens a little, making sure the mixture does not boil.

Add the mushrooms and chicken to the speltotto with the Parmesan and remaining butter, stirring so that all the ingredients are evenly distributed. Serve hot, with a green salad or vegetables of your choice.

500ml/17fl oz/2 cups hot chicken or
vegetable stock.............................
70g/2½oz unsalted butter.................
a drizzle of olive oil.........................
a few thyme sprigs ....
1 garlic clove, bruised ....
200g/7oz wild mushrooms, thinly
sliced ....
4 roasted chicken breasts, bone in
and skin on, shredded, or cooked
chicken, shredded ....
115g/4oz/scant ½ cup crème fraîche...
60g/2¼oz/⅔ cup freshly grated
Parmesan cheese ....
sea salt and freshly ground black
pepper ....
fresh green salad or vegetables,
to serve ....

MOROCCAN LAMB SPELTOTTO

Make the speltotto base with red wine instead of white, and add the harissa paste, cinnamon stick, cumin and garlic with the shallots.

Continue to simmer the speltotto base in the pan, and add the additional hot stock as you did for the speltotto base, waiting for a spoonful to be absorbed before adding more, until all the stock has been absorbed. Simmer for a few more minutes, if necessary, until the pearled spelt is tender.

Add the shredded lamb before the end of cooking so that the meat warms through, and season with salt and pepper. Remove from the heat, stir in a little oil and butter and sprinkle with the parsley. Serve hot with a fresh green salad or vegetables of your choice.

1 tbsp harissa paste ....
1 cinnamon stick................................
1 tsp toasted cumin seeds ....
1 garlic clove, chopped ....
500ml/17fl oz/2 cups hot chicken or
vegetable stock................................
½ recipe quantity cooked lamb shank
meat (see page 128), shredded from
the bone ....
a little olive oil and butter, for
finishing ....
sea salt and freshly ground black
pepper ....
1 handful of herbs, such as parsley......
fresh green salad or vegetables,
to serve ....

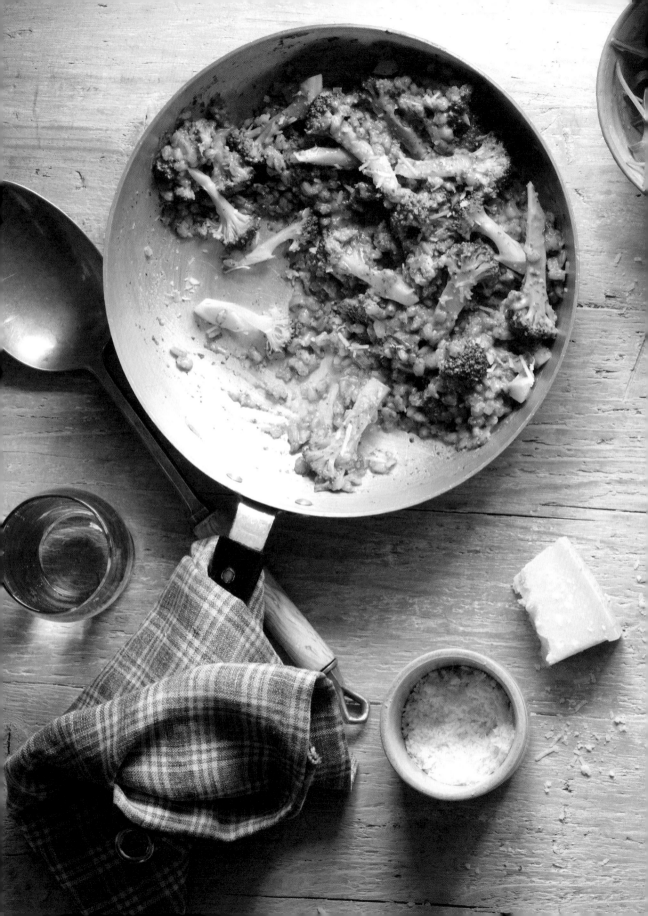

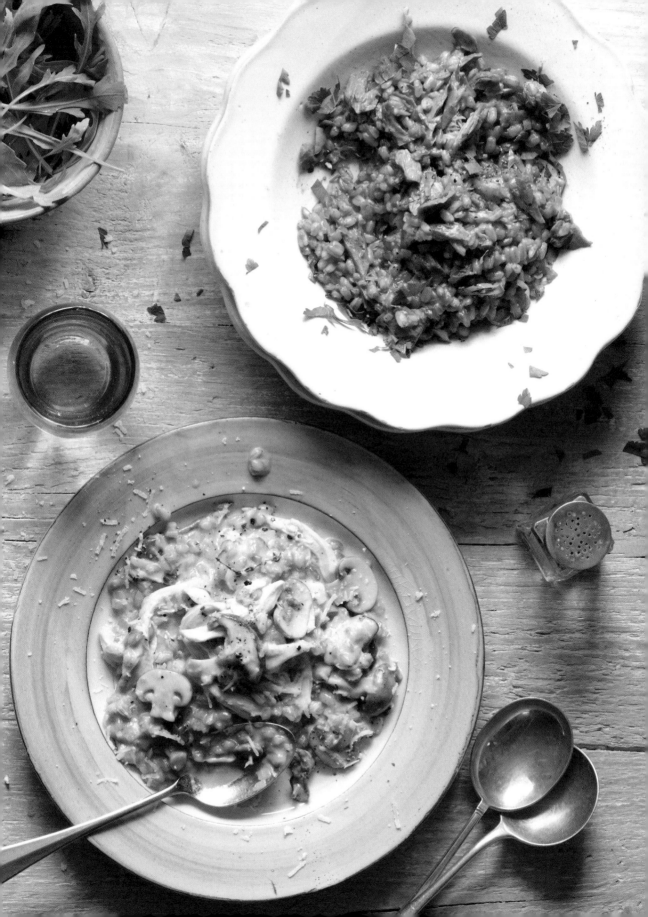

This aromatic and thoroughly delicious fish pie comes from great nutritionist and cook Jessica Andersson. It's quick and easy to prepare and makes a perfect warming supper on a cool autumn or winter's evening.

FISH PIE WITH SPELT CRUMBLE

SERVES 4

PREPARATION TIME: 15 minutes, plus 1 hour chilling COOKING TIME: 25 minutes

Preheat the oven to 200°C/400°F/Gas 6 and lightly grease a deep-sided 20cm/8in square ovenproof dish.

Start by making the crumble topping. Put the flour and salt in a large bowl, then rub in all but 1 tablespoon of the butter and 1 tablespoon of the oil, using your fingertips, until you have a moist crumble. Add more olive oil, if necessary. Add 2 tablespoons of the chopped coriander, the mixed herbs and half the grated cheese and the spelt porridge flakes. Chill in the fridge for 1 hour.

Bring a saucepan of water to the boil over a medium heat. Add the leeks and carrots, reduce the heat and simmer for 5 minutes, or until just tender, then drain.

Meanwhile, mix together all the sauce ingredients, along with the remaining coriander, in a non-metallic bowl. Add the salmon and king prawns and coat well with the mixture. Mix the carrots and leeks with the fish, then spoon the mixture into the prepared dish. Spread the spelt crumble evenly over the top and finish with the remaining grated cheese.

Bake in the oven for 20 minutes, or until the top is crunchy and the salmon is cooked.

When the crumble is almost ready, melt the remaining butter in a large saucepan over a medium heat, add the spinach and cook for a few minutes just until the spinach leaves have all wilted. Season with salt and pepper to taste. Remove the crumble from the oven, sprinkle with extra dill and serve hot with the spinach.

125g/4¼oz butter, diced, plus extra for greasing ....
200g/7oz/1⅔ cups wholegrain spelt flour ....
1 tsp salt...
1–2 tbsp olive oil.................................
1 small bunch coriander leaves, finely chopped..
2 tsp dried mixed herbs ....
140g/5oz/1 cup grated Cheddar cheese ....
100g/3½oz/1 cup spelt porridge flakes ....
2 small leeks, trimmed and sliced ....
2 carrots, diced ....
800g/1lb 12oz salmon, skinned, boned and cut into chunks ....
400g/14oz raw peeled king prawns.....
200g/7oz spinach leaves.....................
sea salt and freshly ground black pepper ....

FOR THE SAUCE:
2 tbsp olive oil...................................
4 tbsp crème fraîche ....
4 tbsp chopped dill leaves, plus extra to garnish ....
2 tsp ground cumin...........................
2 garlic cloves, crushed ....
grated zest of 2 lemons ....
4 tbsp lemon juice ....
2 tsp paprika ....

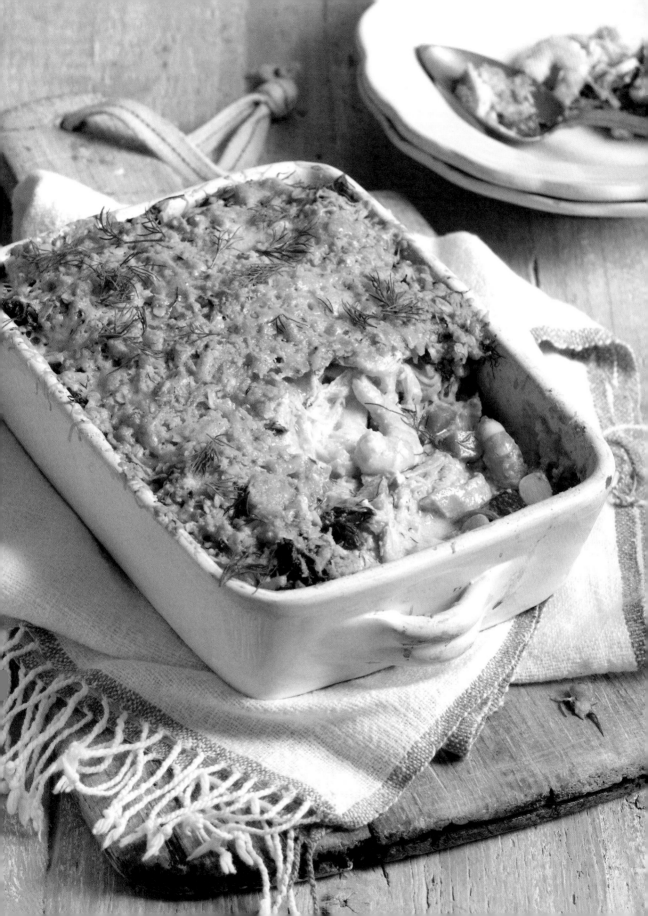

One of our greatest British chefs Mark Hix gave us this fantastic inky pearled spelt recipe and we love the vivid contrast in flavours and colours of this dramatic dish. Mark and I have demonstrated this recipe together in London and in his home town, Lyme Regis, a Dorset coast fishing port. You can buy squid ink in little sachets from any good fishmonger and wild garlic is available online if you cannot find it locally.

PEARLED SPELT & SQUID IN INK & HERBS

SERVES 4

PREPARATION TIME: 15 minutes   COOKING TIME: 20 minutes

Heat the oil in a heavy-based saucepan over a low heat. Add the drained spelt and stir over a low heat for 1–2 minutes until heated through but without allowing it to colour. Add the squid ink and stir well, then begin to add the stock, a little at a time, adding just enough to cover the pearled spelt, then waiting for it to absorb the liquid before adding more, stirring constantly. Continue in this way for about 15 minutes until the pearled spelt is tender and cooked. Stir in two-thirds of the butter and a little more of the stock if the risotto seems a bit too dry; the consistency should be wet but not runny.

Meanwhile, heat the remaining butter in a heavy-based frying pan over a high heat, add the squid and cook for 2–3 minutes, or until just cooked, then stir in the herbs.

Spoon the spelt onto warmed serving plates and scatter the squid over the top to serve.

2 tbsp rapeseed oil

200g/7oz/heaped 1 cup pearled spelt, soaked in cold water for 2 hours, then drained

50g/1¾oz squid ink

1 litre/35fl oz/4 cups fish or vegetable stock

125g/4½oz unsalted butter

150g/5½oz cleaned squid, cut into 2–3cm/¾–1¼in squares

1 tbsp chopped wild or three-cornered garlic, or garlic chives

1 tbsp chopped parsley leaves

1 tbsp chopped chervil leaves

Salting the cod gives it extra flavour and texture, so it holds its shape well when cooking. Try to cook this recipe when asparagus is in season, as the flavours will be sublime. If you grow your own asparagus, so much the better, because it is perfect if you can cook and enjoy it as soon as it is picked.

LEMON & ALMOND COD WITH SPELT & ASPARAGUS

SERVES 4

PREPARATION TIME: 15 minutes, plus 4 hours salting COOKING TIME: 25 minutes

Put the cod in a serving dish and sprinkle evenly with the salt. Cover with cling film and chill in the fridge for 4 hours to salt the cod.

Cook the pearled spelt in boiling water for 20 minutes, or according to the packet instructions. Drain and leave to one side.

Meanwhile rinse the asparagus and snap off the woody ends. Heat the sunflower oil in a saucepan over a medium heat and fry the shallots for a few minutes until soft. Add the chilli and garlic and cook for 2 minutes, then stir in the thyme leaves. Add the white wine, bring to the boil, then simmer for a few minutes until the sauce has reduced by half. Season with salt and pepper and stir in 55g/2oz of the butter, then add the drained pearled spelt and stir so that it is covered in the sauce.

Heat the remaining butter in a frying pan over a medium heat, add the cod and fry for 2–3 minutes on each side until it flakes easily when tested with a fork.

Meanwhile, bring a saucepan of water to the boil over a high heat. Add the asparagus and boil for 1–2 minutes until just tender. Drain well.

Lift the cod onto serving plates, squeeze the lemon juice over the top and sprinkle with the lemon zest and the toasted almonds. Serve with the pearled spelt and asparagus.

4 individual cod fillets ....
1 tbsp sea salt ....
200g/7oz/heaped 1 cup pearled spelt..
400g/14oz asparagus ....
2 tbsp olive oil..................................
2 shallots, chopped...........................
1 green chilli, deseeded and finely
   chopped..
1 garlic clove, chopped ....
1 tsp thyme leaves ....
200ml/7fl oz/scant 1 cup dry white
   wine..
85g/3oz unsalted butter ....
grated zest and juice of ½ lemon ....
75g/2½oz/⅔ cup flaked almonds,
   toasted, or nuts of your choice ....
sea salt and freshly ground black
   pepper ....

The key to great gnocchi is to use the right potato, such as Desirée, and to blend in the flour while the potatoes are hot. The quantity of flour given here is fine for autumn and winter, when floury potatoes are at their peak. In spring and summer, when potatoes are more dense with liquid, you may need 300g/10½oz/2½ cups (or even more) flour to make the dough. The gnocchi will store in an airtight jar in the fridge for up to two weeks.

GNOCCHI WITH WALNUT & BASIL PESTO

SERVES 4

PREPARATION TIME: **30 minutes** COOKING TIME: **1 hour**

Preheat the oven to 180°C/350°F/Gas 4 and lightly flour a baking sheet. Pierce the potatoes several times with a fork. Put them on the sheet and roast for 45 minutes, or until soft and cooked through.

Meanwhile, make the pesto. Put the walnuts and garlic in a food processor and process until finely chopped but still with some texture, so don't over-process. Add the Parmesan and basil and process again. With the motor running, gradually add the oil until the mixture is thick. Season with lemon juice, salt and pepper. Leave to one side.

Remove the potatoes from the oven and, using plastic gloves, quickly remove the potato skins. They can be kept for a snack or discarded.

Put three-quarters of the flour on the work surface and season with the salt. Push the hot potatoes through a potato ricer, or mash them thoroughly, and put on the work surface. Gradually knead the potato into the flour until you have a smooth mixture that isn't too dry. If you find it difficult to bring the dough together, gradually add a little beaten egg to the mixture to help bind the ingredients together, or add more flour, as necessary.

Shape the dough into 2 long sausages about 2.5cm/1in thick and dust them lightly with flour as you go along. Using a sharp knife, slice them into 1.5cm/½in discs, then press them with your thumb into the tines of the fork so they get that characteristic gnocchi shape. Set the gnocchi aside on the prepared baking sheet.

Bring a large saucepan of salted water to the boil over a high heat, add the gnocchi and boil until they rise to the top. Count to 10, then drain. Toss with the walnut pesto and sprinkle with extra Parmesan to serve.

FOR THE GNOCCHI:

200g/7oz/heaped 1½ cups white spelt flour, plus extra for dusting.............
750g/1lb 10oz Desirée potatoes, scrubbed..
¼ tsp sea salt ....
1 egg, beaten (optional).....................

FOR THE WALNUT & BASIL PESTO:

125g/4½oz/scant 1 cup walnuts.........
1 garlic clove, crushed ....
100g/3½oz Parmesan cheese, freshly grated, plus extra to serve................
50g/¾oz basil leaves (a big bunch) .....
100ml/3½fl oz/scant ½ cup extra virgin olive oil................................
juice of ½ small lemon ....
sea salt and freshly ground black pepper ....

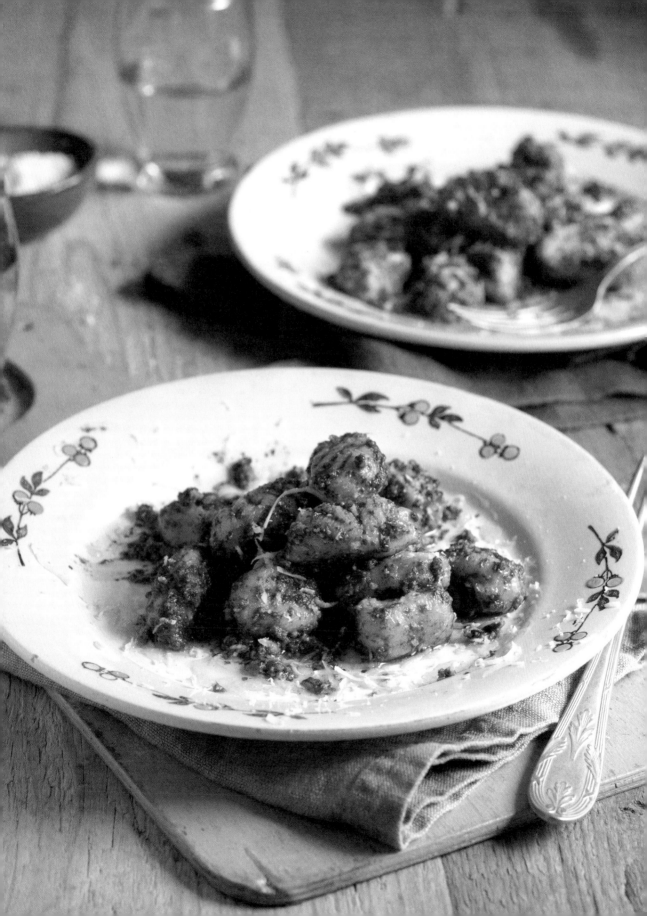

Tagliatelle is a great Italian pasta favourite of mine, originally from the Bologna region where we have spent a lot of time. The pasta can be made in various widths but ideally about 6mm/¼in wide. Refined white spelt makes a lovely pasta, which I much prefer to wholegrain. If you can get hold of them in season, porcini or ceps are a delicious addition. Also, it would be criminal not to add a shaving or two of truffle if you can. I once brought back a few truffles from Florence in my hand luggage and gradually the whole plane smelt very strongly of truffles. However, I didn't learn my lesson and soon the whole fridge stank – not a popular man!

COURGETTE, LEMON, CHILLI & SAFFRON TAGLIATELLE

SERVES 4
PREPARATION TIME: 10 minutes, plus making the pasta COOKING TIME: 10 minutes

Make and roll out the pasta (see page 16), then fold it and cut into strands about 1cm/½in thick.

Heat the oil in a large frying pan over a low heat and fry the shallots for 3–5 minutes until soft. Add the chilli and garlic and cook for a further minute, then add the saffron strands and stir well. Add the courgette slices and continue to cook over a medium heat for 3–5 minutes until the courgette has softened. Add the lemon zest and juice, then drizzle with the oil to create a rich sauce. Stir in the parsley.

Meanwhile, bring a large pan of salted water to the boil, add the tagliatelle and cook for about 3 minutes until al dente. Drain the pasta, then toss with the courgette sauce. Sprinkle with freshly grated Parmesan to serve.

1 recipe quantity Pasta (see page 16)...
2 tbsp sunflower oil ....
2 banana shallots or 6 small shallots,
    finely chopped ....
1 red chilli, deseeded and finely
    chopped...
2 garlic cloves, finely chopped ....
a pinch of saffron strands...................
2 firm courgettes, finely sliced ....
grated zest and juice of 1 lemon ....
2–3 tbsp olive oil...............................
1 bunch of parsley, roughly chopped
freshly grated Parmesan or pecorino
    cheese, for sprinkling ....
sea salt ....

In Italy, everyone has their own version of panzanella, a simple and delicious way to use up stale bread. You start by crisping up the bread so that it is just the right texture. If you only have fresh bread, dry it out for 30 minutes, but if your bread is already stale, just pop the bread cubes in the oven for half the time to bring them back to life. As a variation, you could add some leftover roast vegetables such as butternut squash, aubergine or courgette to this panzanella.

PANZANELLA

SERVES 4
PREPARATION TIME: 20 minutes, plus 20 minutes marinating   COOKING TIME: 30 minutes

Preheat the oven to 150°C/300°F/Gas 2. Put the bread on a large baking sheet and dry out in the oven for 30 minutes for fresh bread or 15 minutes for stale, or until the bread is completely crisp.

Meanwhile, put the red onion slices in a small bowl and just cover with boiling water. Leave to soak while you prepare the rest of the dish.

To make the dressing, whisk together the mustard and vinegar in a large bowl. Gradually pour in the oil, whisking constantly until you have a smooth vinaigrette. Season with the anchovies and pepper.

Remove the bread from the oven and drain the onions.

Squeeze some of the tomato juice into the dressing, then add them to the bowl with the peppers and the drained red onions, dried bread, capers and basil. Toss everything together so the dressing is evenly distributed. Cover with cling film, then leave to marinate at room temperature for 20 minutes before serving so all the flavours infuse into the bread.

Scatter the panzanella on large serving plates and eat while fresh.

1 loaf of white spelt bread, cut into 3cm/1¼in cubes ....
1 small red onion, thinly sliced ....
6 plum tomatoes, quartered ....
1 red pepper, raw or chargrilled, deseeded and cut into chunks ....
1 yellow pepper, raw or chargrilled, deseeded and cut into chunks ....
3 tbsp capers, rinsed and drained ....
1 handful of basil leaves ....

FOR THE MUSTARD & ANCHOVY DRESSING:
1 tsp mustard of your choice ....
3 tbsp white wine vinegar ....
125ml/4fl oz/½ cup olive or rapeseed oil ....
2 salted anchovies, finely chopped ......
freshly ground black pepper ....

My favourite pizza maker is Giuseppe Mascoli, who created Blacks club and the Franco Manca restaurant in London. He is a perfectionist and spent ages trying to get that really fine, crisp base using our spelt flour. He would always want the flour as refined as possible. 'Roger, give me double refined!' So if you are being really picky, sift your flour once more.

PIZZAS

MAKES 6 x 23cm/9in pizzas
PREPARATION TIME: 25 minutes, plus at least 1 hour rising, preferably overnight COOKING TIME: 15 minutes

Lightly oil a large bowl. Put the ingredients in another large bowl and make a well in the centre. Add 430ml/15¼fl oz/1¾ cups lukewarm water and mix together, using a wooden spoon, to a rough dough.

Turn the dough out onto a lightly floured work surface and knead for about 10 minutes, or until the dough is smooth and elastic and springs back when poked. Transfer the kneaded dough to the prepared bowl, cover with a clean, damp tea towel and leave to rise in a warm place for 45 minutes, or until it has doubled in size.

Turn the dough out onto a lightly floured work surface, knock the air out of the dough by punching it with your fist and knead gently once or twice. Shape the dough into 6 evenly sized dough balls, cover again and leave to prove for at least a further 10 minutes. In a perfect scenario, make the dough in the evening and let it rest overnight.

Preheat the oven to 250°C/500°F/Gas 9 and grease several large baking sheets. Roll out the dough pieces to 23cm/9in diameter circles, then put them on the prepared baking sheets. Add your toppings and bake as indicated in the following recipes.

60ml/2fl oz/¼ cup extra virgin olive oil, plus extra for greasing ....
650g/1lb 7oz/5¼ cups white spelt flour, plus extra for dusting ....
1 heaped tsp sea salt ....
15g/½oz/2 tbsp fresh yeast, crumbled, or 7g/¼oz/2 tsp fast-action dried yeast ....
a pinch of sugar.................................
½ tsp dried oregano (optional) ....

TOMATO SAUCE

Heat the sunflower oil in a saucepan over a medium heat. Add the garlic and fry gently for 1 minute until soft but not browned. Stir in the tomatoes, passata, basil, chilli flakes and sugar. Cook for 5–8 minutes until the sauce starts to reduce a little.

Remove from the heat and blend with a hand-held blender until you have a really smooth sauce. Season with a little salt and pepper, then cook over a medium-high heat for a further 5–10 minutes, or until the sauce is quite thick but not solid. Season again, if necessary.

1 tbsp sunflower oil ....
3 garlic cloves, finely chopped ....
400g/14oz/1⅔ cups tinned chopped tomatoes..
500g/1lb 2oz tomato passata ....
1 bunch of basil leaves.......................
½ tsp chilli flakes............................
¼ tsp caster sugar ....
salt and freshly ground black pepper...

TOMATO & MOZZARELLA PIZZA

Spread the tomato sauce over the pizza bases, then spread with the shredded mozzarella. Bake for about 10 minutes until cooked through and bubbling, then drizzle with a little olive oil before serving.

1 recipe quantity Tomato Sauce (see opposite)...
200g/7oz mozzarella cheese, shredded into strips ....
a drizzle of olive oil, to serve..............

FIORENTINA PIZZA

Rinse the spinach in a medium saucepan, then drain the excess liquid away. Put the pan over a medium heat for a few minutes until the spinach has wilted. Season with a grating of nutmeg and a little salt and pepper to taste.

Spread a thin layer of tomato sauce on each of the pizza bases, then spread equal amounts of wilted spinach around each base. Crack an egg on top of each pizza and scatter Parmesan shavings over the whole base. Season with a little black pepper. Bake for 10 minutes until cooked through and bubbling. Drizzle with a little olive oil to serve.

250g/9oz spinach leaves.....................
a pinch of freshly grated nutmeg ....
100g/3½oz Tomato Sauce (see opposite)...
6 eggs ....
50g/1¾oz Parmesan cheese, shaved into strips ....
sea salt and freshly ground black pepper ....
a drizzle of olive oil, to serve..............

PORK & FENNEL MEATBALL PIZZA

Make the meatballs to the end of step 3 of the Pork & Fennel Meatballs recipe (see page 131) so you have uncooked bite-sized meatballs.

Spread the pizza bases with tomato sauce, then top with the uncooked meatballs and sprinkle with the mozzarella. Season with salt and pepper. Bake for 8–10 minutes until puffed up, golden and the meatballs are cooked. Top with some Parmesan shavings and serve with a handful of rocket.

1 recipe quantity Pork & Fennel Meatballs (see page 131) ....
1 recipe quantity Tomato Sauce (see opposite)...
200g/7oz mozzarella cheese, shredded
a few Parmesan shavings.....................
sea salt and freshly ground black pepper ....
rocket leaves or herbs, to serve............

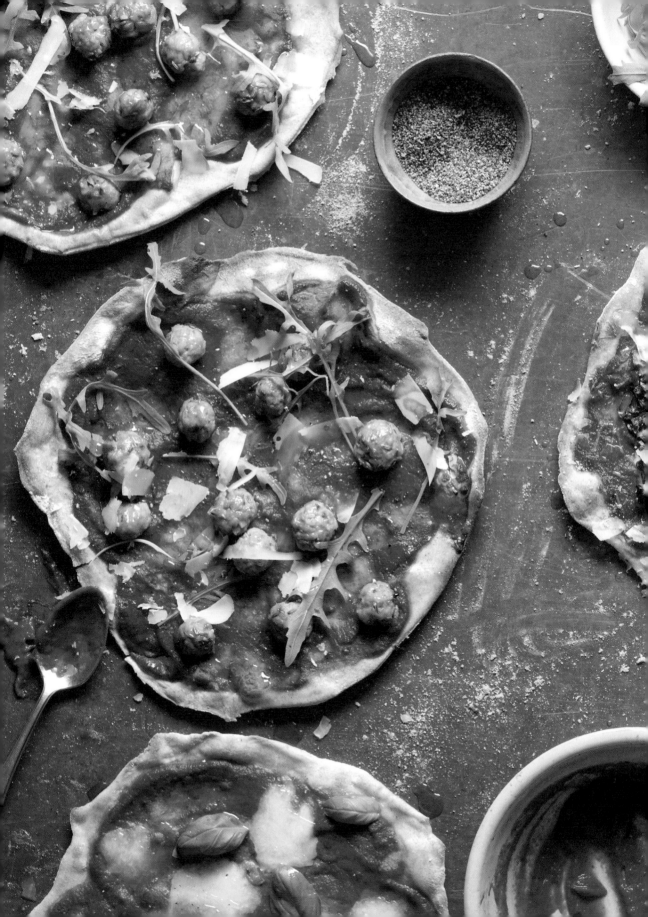

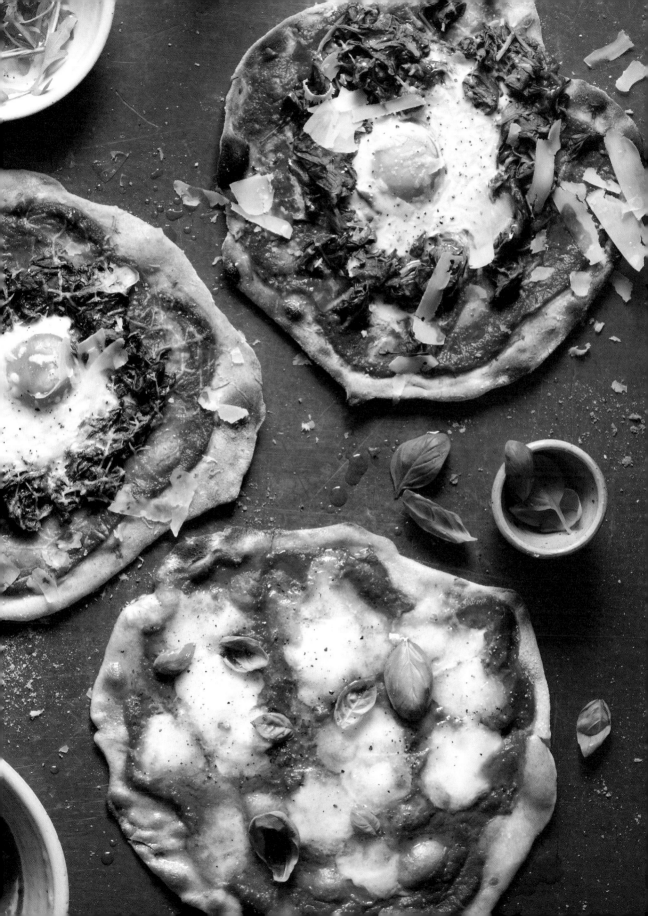

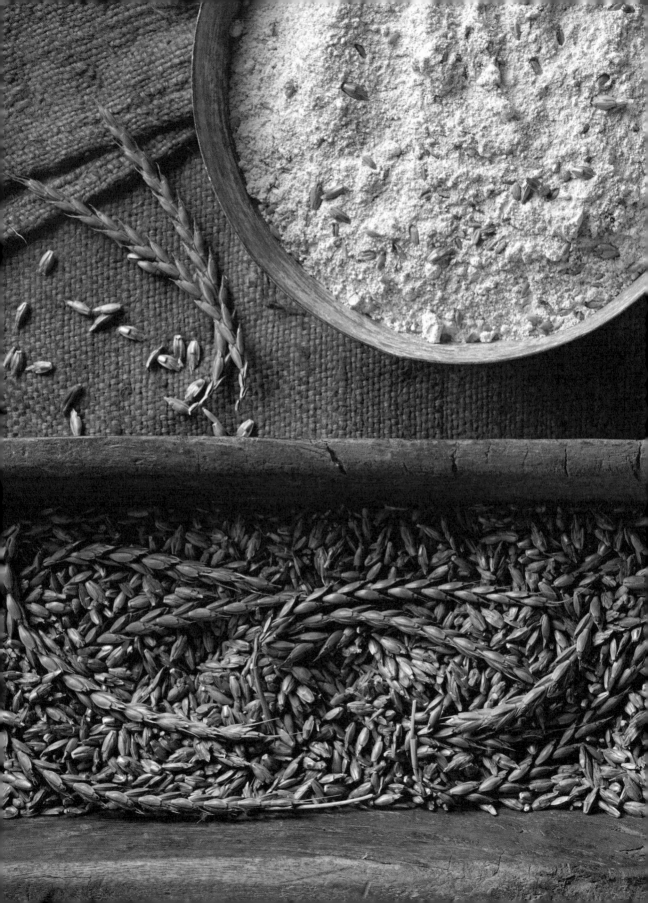

DESSERTS

Puddings, deuxièmes, sweets, desserts – it doesn't really matter what you call them, they are that last fanfare of surprise with which to indulge your guests. It is funny how in Britain if you eat too much at the dining table we will refer to you as a 'greedy pig', whereas in Italy you are lorded with the title '*buona forchetta*', which means you're a 'good fork' and love your food.

I have to admit to having a sweet tooth – definitely a *buona forchetta*, quite possibly a greedy pig – and during the journey of writing this book, have enjoyed testing every one of the recipes in this chapter. Fruit is often a key feature in desserts, and as a source of natural sugars, we have tried to use as much as we can. I'm a great fan of the simple 'pudding cake', and Blackberry Pudding (see page 156) is an easy one to make. Also, try Autumn Fruit Grumbles (see page 158). My wife is known to our best friends as 'Queen of the Crumble' (mainly because it's the only pud that she can't destroy and they get served it very regularly! ... I can feel that frying pan hovering!). She adds our spelt muesli to the topping for added crunch.

One of my real favourites is Spelt Cranachan (see page 154). You don't have to be able to pronounce it, but do have a go at making this classic Scottish Gaelic dessert.

For those of you who haven't come across cranachan before, it is a Scottish Gaelic dessert that sounds a handful but is absolutely delicious. Originally it was a summer dish eaten around harvest time. There is a tale that says if you put a ring in the mixture and serve it at a wedding, whoever finds the ring in their dish will be the next to marry. Quite what happens if you are already married, I am not sure!

SPELT CRANACHAN

SERVES 4

PREPARATION TIME: 10 minutes, plus making and cooling the porridge

Put the cream, honey and whisky in a large bowl and whisk, using an electric whisk, until soft peaks form.

Spoon a layer of the spelt porridge into tall glasses, then a layer of the poached raspberries and finally the flavoured cream. Sprinkle with the spelt porridge flakes, if using. Chill in the fridge until you are ready to serve.

700ml/24fl oz/generous 2¾ cups
double cream ....
2 tbsp clear honey ....
3½ tbsp malt whisky ....
70g/2½oz cooked and cooled
Porridge (see page 49).....................
200g/7oz poached raspberries or other
poached or fresh fruit of your choice
1 tbsp spelt porridge flakes, toasted
(optional) ....

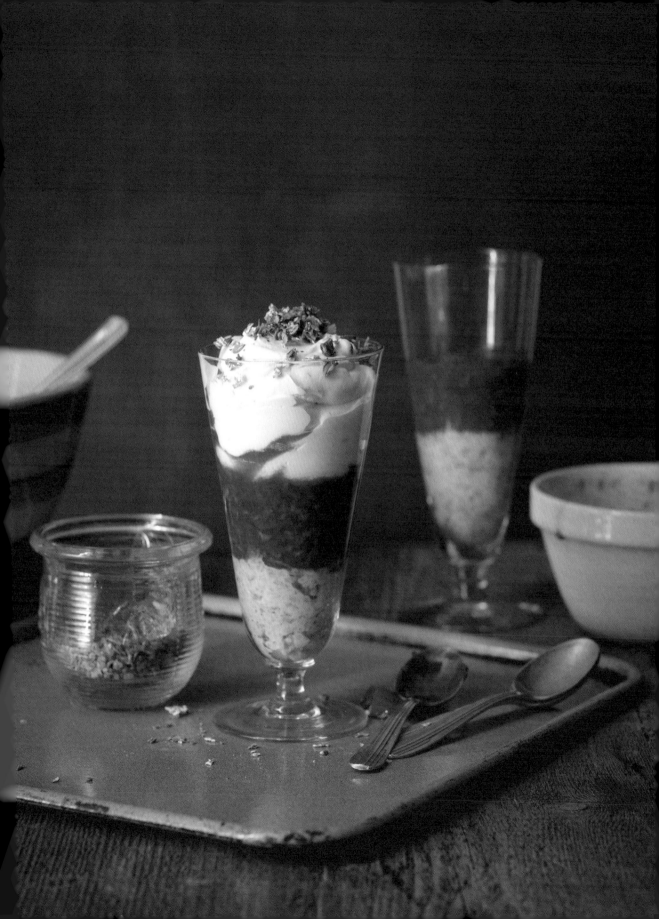

This is a really easy 'pudding cake' that is perfect for entertaining as it is one that can be rustled up in minutes, allowing you to get on with the more important task of having a good time with your guests. The blackberries lend an inky, perfumed sweetness to the pudding but you could, of course, use mixed summer berries or chopped rhubarb instead.

BLACKBERRY PUDDING

SERVES 8
PREPARATION TIME: 15 minutes COOKING TIME: 50 minutes

Preheat the oven to 180°C/350°F/Gas 4 and lightly grease a 30 x 20cm/ 12 x 8in cake tin or ceramic roasting dish.

Spread the blackberries over the base of the prepared tin and sprinkle with the lemon zest and juice, stirring a little so that the juice mixes with the berries.

Whisk the eggs, caster sugar and vanilla in a large bowl for 5 minutes, or until light and fluffy. Sift the flour, ground almonds, baking powder and salt into a medium bowl. Gradually add the flour mixture to the egg mixture alternately with the melted butter and soured cream. Fold the mixture together until you have a smooth, thick batter.

Scoop the batter over the blackberries and sprinkle the demerara sugar over the top for extra crunch.

Bake for 45–50 minutes, or until the pudding looks golden brown and a skewer inserted in the centre comes out clean. Bear in mind that if there is some blackberry on the skewer this is normal, so just insert the skewer halfway down into the pudding to check the batter is cooked.

Transfer to a wire rack to cool a little, then serve warm, with crème fraîche, or ice cream of your choice.

125g/4½oz unsalted butter, melted and cooled, plus extra for greasing ...
400g/14oz fresh blackberries ....
grated zest and juice of 1 lemon ....
3 large eggs ....
200g/7oz/scant 1 cup golden caster sugar ....
1 tsp vanilla extract ....
150g/5½oz/scant 1¼ cups white spelt flour ....
55g/2oz/heaped ½ cup ground almonds ....
1 tsp baking powder ....
¼ tsp fine sea salt ....
125ml/4fl oz/½ cup soured cream ......
2 tbsp demerara sugar ....
crème fraîche or ice cream, to serve .....

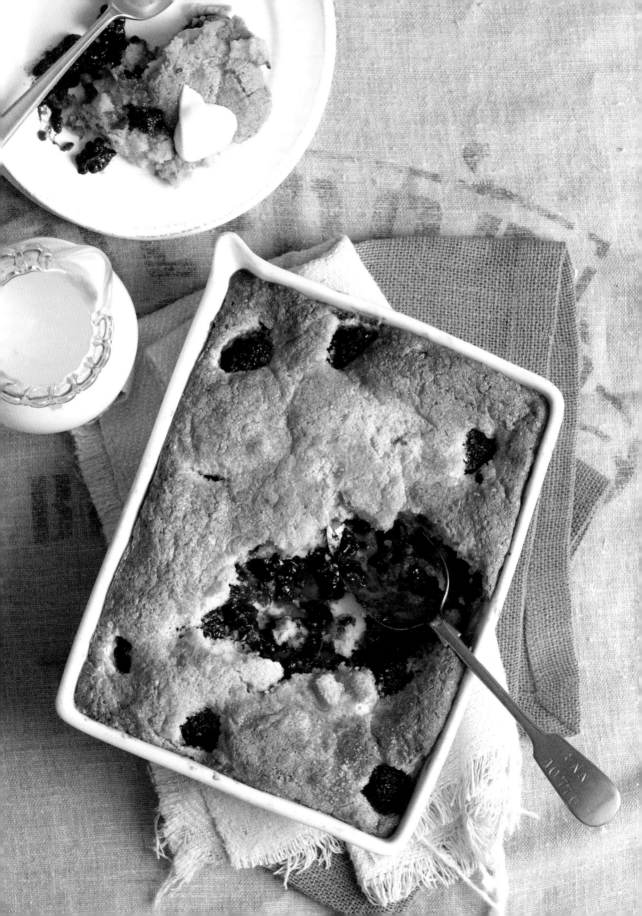

This is my wife Monty's marvellous invention, a classic berry crumble/granola hybrid. If you can go blackberry picking in late summer, then nothing beats a wild blackberry grumble (unless you are lucky enough to have autumn-flowering raspberries as well). Monty mixes the two for a great colour, and if she has a stray banana or two, then they'll be thinly sliced to make a delicious base. These grumbles can be made in individual ramekins or in a large dish.

AUTUMN FRUIT GRUMBLES

SERVES 6

PREPARATION TIME: 20 minutes, plus 1 hour chilling COOKING TIME: 20 minutes

Put the flour in a large bowl, then rub in the butter, using your fingertips, until the mixture resembles fine breadcrumbs. Stir in the sugar and the granola. Chill in the fridge for 1 hour or put in the freezer for 30 minutes for an extra-crisp grumble topping.

Preheat the oven to 180°C/350°F/Gas 4 and grease a 30 x 20cm/12 x 8in deep ovenproof dish or 6 individual ramekins.

If you are going for the banana option, put a few slices in the bottom of the dish or dishes. Pack the berries on top, adding sugar to taste if your berries need sweetening. Cover the berries with the chilled grumble topping.

Put the dish on a baking sheet and bake for 20 minutes, or until the grumble is golden in colour and crisp to the touch, and the berry juice is erupting. Monty says that a grumble looks like a mini Mount Vesuvius when baking in the oven – bubbling and spitting with inky berry juice.

Serve with crème fraîche, clotted cream or ice cream.

175g/6oz/heaped 1⅓ cups white spelt flour or a mixture of white and wholegrain spelt flour ....
115g/4oz unsalted butter, diced, plus extra for greasing ....
115g/4oz/scant ⅔ cup light soft brown sugar.....................................
115g/4oz Farmhouse Granola (see page 46).....................................
1 banana, sliced (optional).................
500g/1lb 2oz mixed berries, such as blackberries, raspberries, blueberries, whatever takes your fancy ....
sugar or sweetener of your choice (optional) ....
crème fraîche, clotted cream or ice cream, to serve ....

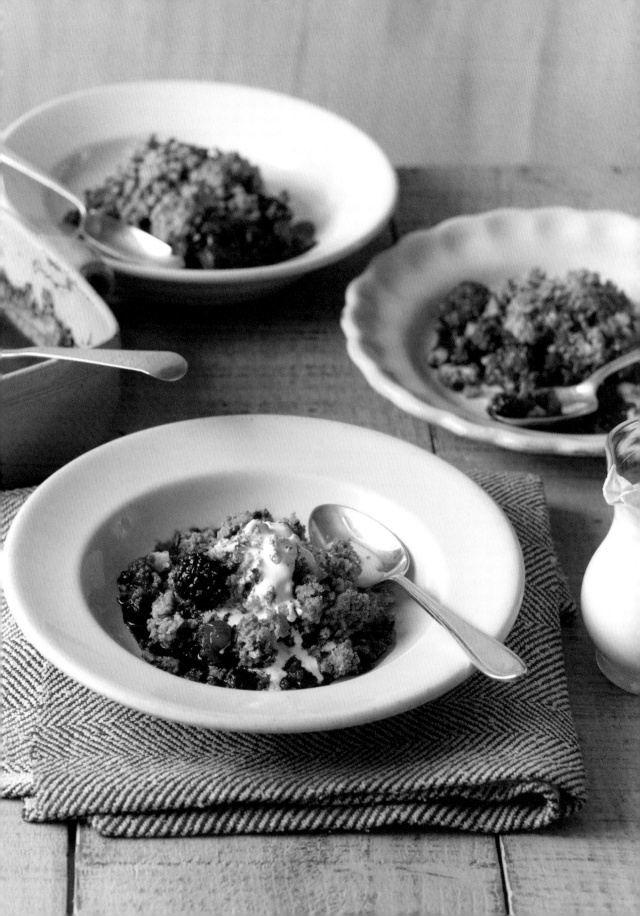

This makes another great dish for entertaining as you can prepare it in advance, then assemble it at the last minute. Keep the curd in the fridge and it will last for several weeks, while the shortbread can be kept in an airtight tin.

LEMON & ORANGE CURD WITH VANILLA SHORTBREAD

SERVES 6
PREPARATION TIME: 15 minutes, plus 2 hours chilling COOKING TIME: 25 minutes

Heat the lemon and orange zest and juice, the butter and sugar in a saucepan over a low heat until the butter has completely melted. Whisk the egg yolks in a separate bowl until fluffy. Add to the juice mixture and whisk until thick. Pass through a sieve into serving dishes and chill for at least 2 hours.

Meanwhile, to make the shortbread, put the flour in a bowl, then rub in the butter, using your fingertips, until the mixture resembles breadcrumbs. Stir in the sugar and vanilla seeds and mix to a fairly stiff dough. Roll out the dough into a fat sausage, wrap in cling film and leave to rest in the fridge for 1 hour.

Preheat the oven to 160°C/315°F/Gas 2–3 and lightly grease a large baking sheet.

Slice the chilled dough into 1cm/½in thick discs and put them on the prepared baking sheet. Bake for 20 minutes, or until golden in colour and slightly sandy to the touch. Don't let the shortbread brown.

Transfer carefully to a wire rack and sprinkle with sugar while still hot, then leave to cool.

To assemble the dessert, put a biscuit on a plate and scoop or pipe the citrus curd on top. You can top with another shortbread, if you wish.

FOR THE LEMON & ORANGE CURD:
grated zest and juice of ½ lemon ....
grated zest and juice of ½ orange........
90g/3¼oz unsalted butter...................
80g/2¾oz/⅓ cup caster sugar ....
3 egg yolks.......................................

FOR THE VANILLA SHORTBREAD:
150g/5½oz/scant 1¼ cups white spelt flour ....
100g/3½oz unsalted butter, diced, plus extra for greasing ....
50g/1¾oz/scant ¼ cup caster sugar, plus extra for sprinkling..................
¼ vanilla pod, seeds scraped out.........
a little oil, for greasing.......................

Lemon tart is a classic, and not to be messed with. The only tweak we have made is using spelt flour for the pastry, which adds that slightly nutty flavour. Always try to buy unwaxed lemons but if you can't get them, make sure you scrub the lemons before you start.

LEMON TART

SERVES 6
PREPARATION TIME: 10 minutes, plus making the pastry case and 30 minutes cooling
COOKING TIME: 1½ hours

Preheat the oven to 180°C/350°F/Gas 4 and lightly grease a 23cm/9in tart tin.

Make the pastry, roll it out on a lightly floured surface and use to line the prepared tin and bake blind (see page 14). Sit the tin on a baking sheet and leave to cool completely. Turn the oven down to 150°C/300°F/Gas 2.

Meanwhile, put the eggs and sugar in a large bowl and beat together for a few seconds until the ingredients are evenly blended. Add the remaining ingredients and stir together, then pour the mixture into the cooled pastry case.

Carefully put the tart, on the baking sheet, in the oven and bake for 50–60 minutes until the filling is set but still has a slight wobble when you nudge it. Transfer to a wire rack to cool.

1 recipe quantity Shortcrust Pastry (see page 14)....................................

6 eggs ....

225g/8oz/scant 1 cup golden caster sugar..

grated zest and juice of 6 small lemons...

125ml/4 fl oz/½ cup double cream.....

Pecan pie is an American export that we gratefully receive. Traditionally a Thanksgiving dish, our spelt pastry crust combines perfectly to reflect the flavour of this sweet nut. And for my version, I've added a slug of rum.

PECAN PIE

SERVES 6
PREPARATION TIME: 15 minutes, plus making the pastry case and 10 minutes cooling
COOKING TIME: 45 minutes

Preheat the oven to 180°C/350°F/Gas 4 and lightly grease a 23cm/9in pie tin.

Make the pastry, roll it out on a lightly floured surface and use to line the prepared tin and bake blind (see page 14). Sit the tin on a baking sheet and leave to cool completely. Turn the oven down to 170°C/325°F/Gas 3.

Put the eggs in a large bowl and lightly whisk, then add all the remaining ingredients except the pecans. Crush two-thirds of the pecans and reserve 100g/3½oz/1 cup of pecan halves.

Add the crushed pecans to the large bowl with the other filling ingredients and mix well. Pour this into the prepared pie tin, arrange the pecan halves on top of the filling and bake for 45 minutes, or until the filling has set. Transfer to a wire rack to cool slightly before serving.

1 recipe quantity Shortcrust Pastry (see page 14) ....
a little flour, for dusting ....
3 eggs ....
200g/7oz/scant 1¼ cups dark soft brown sugar ....
125g/4oz/scant ½ cup golden syrup ...
75g/2½oz unsalted butter, melted and cooled ....
2 tbsp golden or dark rum ....
1 tsp vanilla extract ....
250g/9oz/2½ cups pecan halves ....

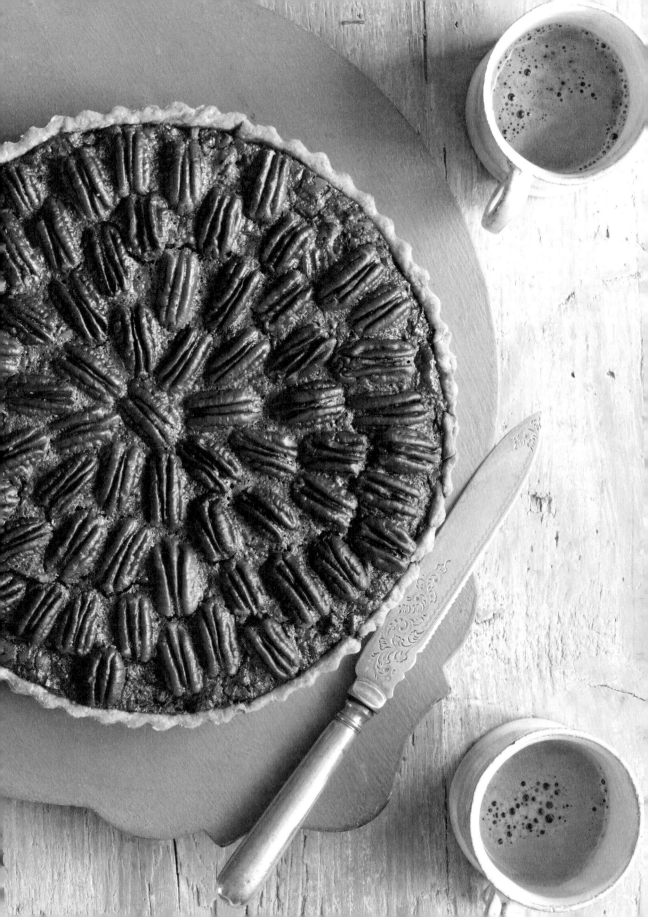

What is not to love about sticky toffee puddings – apart from the regrettable fact that we can only enjoy them in moderation! This is one of those naughty recipes that we all deserve occasionally because they are just such a treat. It is also a really useful dessert, as the puddings can be made in advance, wrapped tightly in cling film, then labelled and frozen, ready to emerge and delight your guests.

STICKY TOFFEE PUDDINGS

SERVES 8

PREPARATION TIME: 15 minutes   COOKING TIME: 30 minutes for individual puddings, 50 minutes for a large pudding

Preheat the oven to 180°C/350°F/Gas 4 and grease eight 185ml/6fl oz/ ¾ cup pudding moulds, or a large ovenproof dish.

Put the dates, treacle, bicarbonate of soda and 250ml/9fl oz/1 cup cold water in a saucepan and bring to the boil. Remove from the heat and blend, using a hand-held blender or a blender, until completely smooth.

Beat together the butter and sugar, using an electric whisk, until pale and fluffy. Add the eggs one at a time, including a spoonful of the flour with each egg to prevent the mixture from splitting, beating well between each addition. Add the puréed date mixture, fold in the remaining flour and combine using a figure of eight motion with a large metal spoon or spatula. Don't beat the mixture or it will be tough.

Pour the mixture into the prepared moulds, filling about two-thirds full so that they have ample room to rise while baking. Bake for 20–30 minutes for individual puddings or 40–50 minutes for one large pudding until well risen and springy to the touch. Although the puddings are dark in colour, you will see that they also brown a little. Remove from the oven and leave to cool for 5–10 minutes before serving. (If you are going to use them another time, turn them out onto a wire rack and allow them to cool completely before wrapping and chilling.)

Meanwhile to make the sticky toffee sauce, put all the ingredients except the cream in a saucepan and bring to the boil. Remove from the heat and fold in the cream. Pour over the puddings and serve with a little extra pouring cream for an extra-indulgent dessert.

FOR THE PUDDINGS:

50g/1¾oz unsalted butter, softened, plus extra for greasing ....

175g/6oz/scant 1¼ cups chopped pitted dates ....

1½ tsp black treacle ....

1½ tsp bicarbonate of soda ....

185g/6½oz/1 cup dark soft brown sugar...

2 large eggs, lightly beaten ....

175g/6oz/1⅓ cups white spelt flour....

1 tsp baking powder ....

FOR THE STICKY TOFFEE SAUCE:

75g/2½oz unsalted butter..................

75g/2½oz/scant ¼ cup golden syrup

75g/2½oz/heaped ⅓ cup dark soft brown sugar...................................

80ml/2½fl oz/⅓ cup double cream, plus extra to serve ....

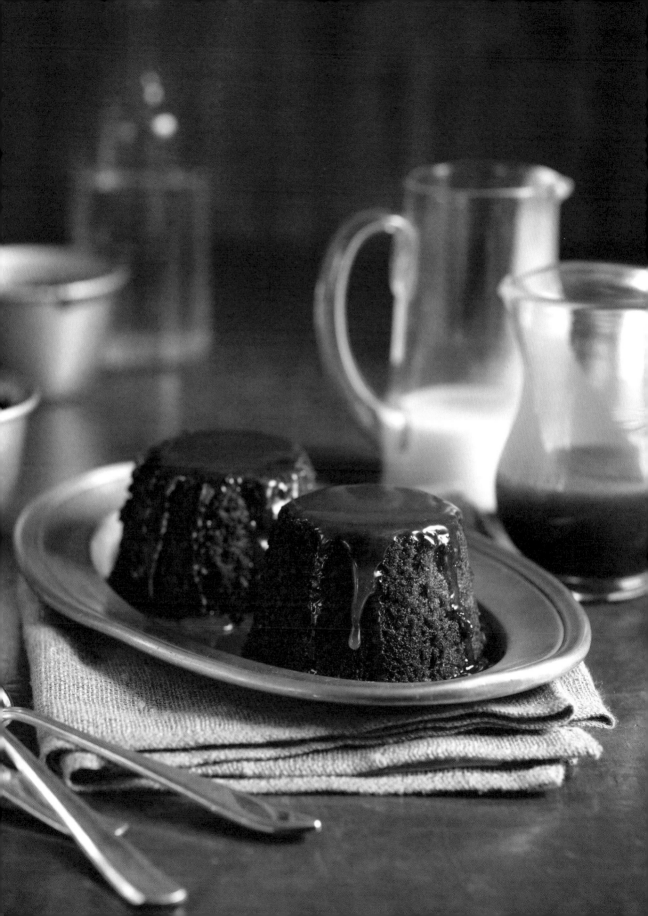

Choux pastry never fails to impress, and it's easy once you get the hang of it. It's a classic with good reason, because these light and pillowy little buns can be topped and filled with any number of delicious sauces, curds, fruit, chocolate – whatever takes your fancy.

CHOUX BUNS

SERVES 4

PREPARATION TIME: 25 minutes, plus 10 minutes cooling COOKING TIME: 35 minutes

Preheat the oven to 200°C/400°F/Gas 6 and line a baking sheet with baking paper. Fold a sheet of baking paper in half so that it has a crease running down the middle and then open it out again.

Put 210ml/7½fl oz/generous ¾ cup water and the butter in a medium saucepan over a low heat and bring to a simmer, stirring to make sure that the butter has melted completely before the water reaches the boil.

While the water is heating up, sift the flour and salt together onto the baking paper and repeat twice. This is to aerate the flour. Once the water is boiling, use the baking paper to make a funnel and shoot the flour and salt into the boiling water and butter mixture. Immediately turn off the heat and stir the mixture vigorously for about 20 seconds until it is thick and comes away from the side of the pan.

Spread the dough on a plate and leave to cool for 10 minutes to room temperature, then put the dough back in the saucepan but keep it off the heat. Gradually add the beaten eggs and make sure that you really beat the mixture each time to fully incorporate the egg. Do this until the mixture reaches a smooth, dropping consistency.

Use two teaspoons to put little balls of choux dough on the prepared baking sheets, leaving a space between each one.

Bake on the top shelf of the oven for 15–20 minutes until puffed up and golden. It is important not to open the oven door for the first 10 minutes, as this can lead to the collapse of the choux buns.

Remove the buns from the oven, insert a skewer underneath each bun and hollow out any uncooked choux mixture before placing them back in the oven for 5–10 minutes to completely dry out. Transfer to a wire rack to cool, then fill and glaze, as you like.

85g/3oz unsalted butter, diced...........
115g/4oz/scant 1 cup white spelt flour ....
a pinch of salt....................................
3 large eggs, lightly beaten.................

CREAM FILLING & BERRY GLAZE

Sift the icing sugar into a bowl and add the berry juice a little at a time, mixing with a wooden spoon until it forms a glaze. Cover with cling film and leave to one side until you are ready to ice the buns.

Cut open the side of the buns. Whip the cream until it forms soft peaks, then spoon it into a piping bag with a large, plain nozzle and pipe into the choux buns. Top with a few of the berries, then close the lids. Pile onto a plate and spoon over the berry glaze.

200g/7oz/1⅔ cups icing sugar, sifted..

4 tbsp fresh mixed berry juice, strained..

300ml/10fl oz/scant 1¼ cups double cream...

100g/3½oz mixed berries ....

CHOCOLATE GANACHE

Put 150g/5½oz of the chocolate, the double cream and salt in a heatproof bowl set over a saucepan of gently simmering water and leave to melt without stirring. Remove from the heat.

Beat the ganache, using an electric whisk, for a few minutes until it is light and fluffy. Spoon it into a piping bag with a large, plain nozzle and pipe it into the choux buns. Meanwhile, grate about 1 tablespoon of the remaining chocolate and melt the remainder in a small heatproof bowl over a saucepan of hot water. Dip the top of each bun into the melted chocolate and sprinkle with the grated chocolate.

200g/7oz dark chocolate (70% cocoa solids), chopped...........................

125ml/4fl oz/½ cup double cream......

a pinch of sea salt ....

PASSION FRUIT CURD

Cut the passion fruit in half and scoop out the seeds and juicy flesh into a small blender. Pulse briefly to separate the seeds from the flesh, then rub the juice and flesh through a sieve into a bowl. Reserve half the seeds for folding through the finished curd.

Put the passion fruit flesh in a large bowl with the caster sugar, eggs and egg yolks, and stir until thick. Melt the butter in a saucepan over a low heat. Add the passion fruit mixture, stirring continuously and making sure it doesn't come to the boil or the eggs will scramble. Cook for 5–8 minutes, stirring, until the mixture coats the back of a wooden spoon. Add the reserved passion fruit seeds and stir through.

Spoon the curd into a bowl, cover and chill in the fridge. Once you're ready, spoon the curd into a piping bag with a large, plain nozzle and pipe it into the hole in the bottom of the choux buns. Sift over the icing sugar to serve. You can keep any extra passion fruit curd in an airtight container in the fridge for a few weeks.

12 ripe passion fruit ....

115g/4oz/½ cup golden caster sugar...

2 eggs ....

2 egg yolks..

140g/5oz unsalted butter...................

a pinch of sea salt ....

a little icing sugar, for dusting............

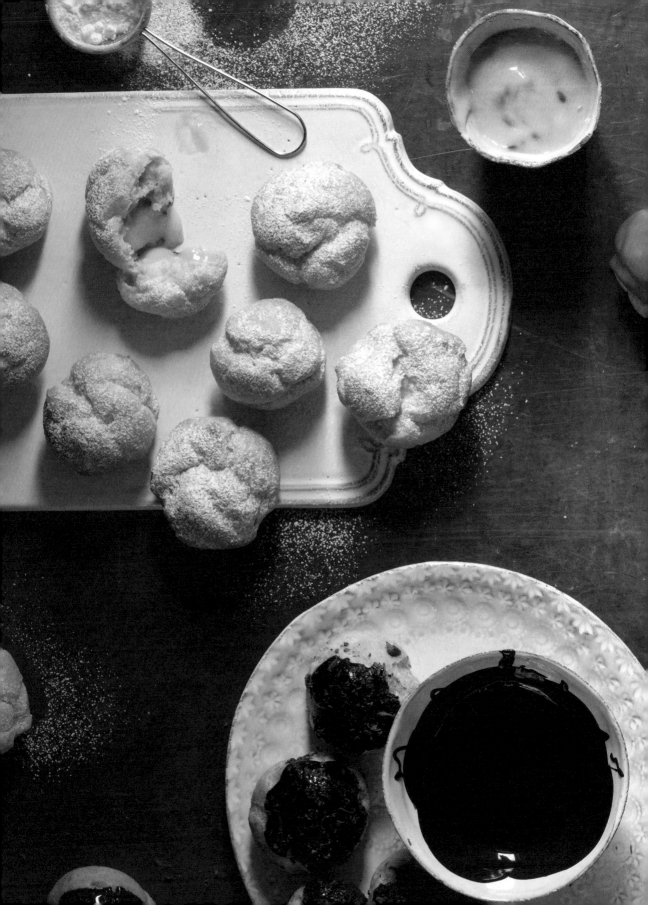

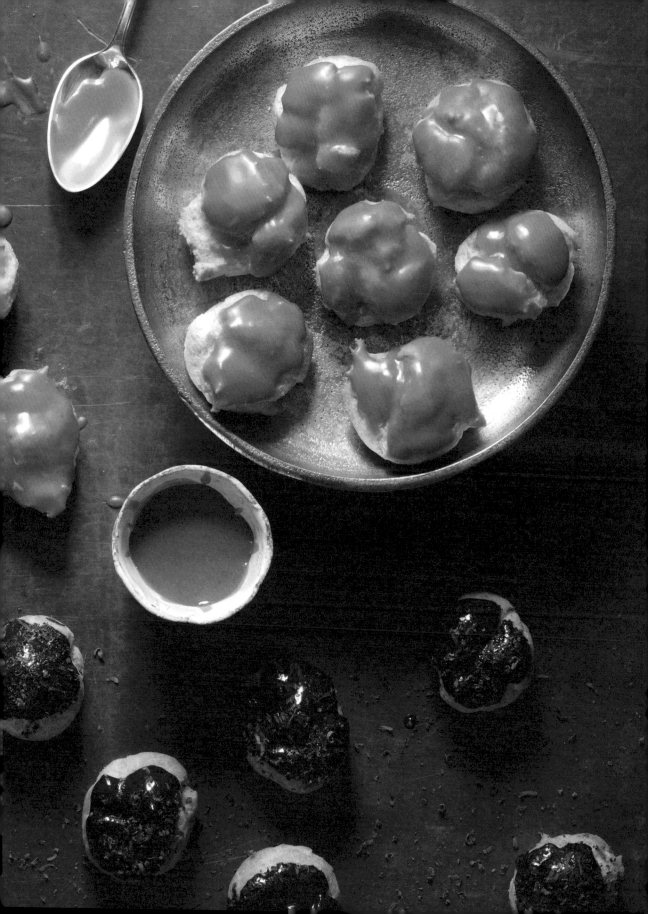

I am proud to say that this is a very English recipe and dates back to medieval times, though you don't want to know the original ingredients! My childhood memory is a silver sixpence inserted in the pie and lots of burning rum on top! Suffice to say that spelt makes it a very special pudding.

CHRISTMAS PUDDING

SERVES: 4

PREPARATION TIME: 20 minutes, plus 2 hours standing, then cooling and storing COOKING TIME: 8 hours

Put all the ingredients up to and including the cinnamon in a large bowl. Stir in the melted butter, eggs and juice and mix well. Cover and leave to stand at room temperature for at least 2 hours or preferably overnight.

Grease the sides of a 1 litre/35fl oz/4 cup pudding basin and cut two circles of baking paper to fit the diameter of the top of the basin.

Give the pudding mixture another stir, then scoop it into the prepared basin. Cover the top of the pudding with the baking paper circles, then spread kitchen foil over the top of the pudding basin, tucking it in really well around the outer rim of the basin.

Place the pudding basin in a large saucepan, then fill the pan with water until the water reaches halfway up the basin. Put the lid on the saucepan and bring to the boil, then simmer for 5 hours, topping up with boiling water as necessary.

Carefully remove the pudding and cool it on a wire rack. Be sure to leave the foil and baking paper on as the pudding cools. Store the pudding in a cool, dark place until required.

When you're ready to eat the pudding, remove and refresh the greaseproof and foil layers. Put the basin in a saucepan again and fill the pan with water until it reaches halfway up the basin. Cover, bring to the boil, then boil, as before, for a further 3 hours. Invert the pudding onto a warm serving plate and serve warm, with brandy butter, cream or other accompaniment of your choice. Flambéing the pudding with brandy when serving is traditional, some would say mandatory!

150g/5½oz/scant 1¼ cups raisins.......
150g/5½oz/scant 1¼ cups sultanas ....
100g/3½oz/heaped ¾ cup currants ....
55g/2oz/heaped ⅓ cup pitted dates or prunes, chopped ....
55g/2oz/⅓ cup chopped mixed peel...
30g/1oz/2 tbsp blanched almonds......
100g/3½oz/heaped ¾ cup wholegrain spelt flour ....
55g/2oz/¼ cup caster sugar ....
finely grated zest of 1 lemon ....
1 tsp mixed spice ....
1 tsp ground cinnamon ....
75g/2½oz unsalted butter, melted and cooled...
2 eggs, lightly beaten ....
3 tbsp orange juice (or fruit juice of choice)..
brandy butter and cream, to serve.......

Everyone loves ice cream, and this is a riff on classic brown bread ice cream. The slight crunch of the caramelized breadcrumbs adds texture and extra flavour to what is otherwise an elegant, simple ice cream recipe. If you like the flavour of rum or whisky you could add a couple of tablespoons of either to the custard base for an extra kick.

BROWN BREAD ICE CREAM

SERVES 4

PREPARATION TIME: 15 minutes, plus cooling and churning COOKING TIME: 30 minutes

Preheat the oven to 180°C/350°F/Gas 4 and line a baking tray with baking paper.

Blitz the bread in a blender until you have coarse breadcrumbs. Add the melted butter and demerara sugar and blitz again. Spread this on the prepared baking tray and bake for 15–20 minutes until the breadcrumbs are crisp and golden brown. Remove from the oven and leave to cool completely. Store in an airtight container until you are ready to churn the ice cream.

Meanwhile, to make the ice cream custard base, bring the milk and cream just to the boil in a saucepan over a medium-high heat. Allow to cool for a few minutes until tepid. Put the egg yolks and brown sugar in a medium bowl, stir together, then add the vanilla and salt. Rinse out the saucepan in which you scalded the milk and cream, then return the custard base to this pan. Put over a gentle heat and stir continuously with a wooden spoon for 5–8 minutes until the custard coats the back of the wooden spoon. Sieve any scrambled egg bits out of the custard, if need be, and allow to cool completely, ideally overnight, before churning the ice cream.

When you're ready to churn the ice cream, mix in the crisp spelt breadcrumbs and churn according to the instructions on the ice cream machine. Alternatively, freeze the mixture in a suitable container for 2 hours, then break up the ice crystals with a fork and return it to the freezer. Repeat this twice more, then leave to freeze.

3 slices of stale Sharpham Park Farmhouse Loaf (see page 20).........

75g/2½oz unsalted butter, melted and cooled...

55g/2oz/¼ cup demerara sugar...........

500ml/17fl oz/2 cups full-fat milk......

300ml/10½fl oz/scant 1¼ cups double cream ....

6 egg yolks...

150g/5½oz/heaped ¾ cup light soft brown sugar....................................

1 tsp vanilla extract...........................

¼ tsp sea salt ....

INDEX

ACKNOWLEDGEMENTS

A huge thank you for all of the spelt recipes sent to me and Sharpham Park over the years. As I'm sure you'll appreciate, there are too many to thank everyone separately, but we've enjoyed using them to experiment with this wonderfully versatile grain.

And thanks to all the people who have helped and supported me.

Signe Johansen – without whom I couldn't have put this book together.

My family, particularly Monty and Freddie, both of whom have valiantly coped with me creating my spelt world and making it a better place!

Two great nutritionists, Amanda Hamilton and Jessica Andersson, who have given me lots of sage advice, and helped me to compile the nutrition information.

Our Sharpham Park team; led by the ever-patient Paula Gledhill, my PAs Hayley Philp and Catie Watson, the catering team led by Julieanne Fenemer, Elliot Leigh and Annie Morgan.

The list of chefs, bakers, food writers and suppliers who have given us recipes, checked recipes and given enormous support: Annie Bell, Sven-Hanson Britt, Gennaro Contaldo, Gizzi Erskine, Adam Fellows, Alex Gooch, Rachel Green, Trine Hahnemann, Angela Hartnett, Tom Hitchmough, Mark Hix, Edd Kimber, Brendan Lynch, David Marshall, Tommi Miers, Phil Nicodemi, Sam Ross, Yottam Ottolenghi, Mary Thomas.

My agent, Tom Williams.

Last, but certainly not least, the Nourish team, led by Grace Cheetham, but particularly Rebecca Woods and Georgie Hewitt, who nurtured me through the process.

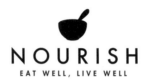

NOURISH
EAT WELL, LIVE WELL

Here at Nourish we're all about wellbeing through food and drink – irresistible dishes with a serious good-for-you factor. If you want to eat and drink delicious things that set you up for the day, suit any special diets, keep you healthy and make the most of the ingredients you have, we've got some great ideas to share with you. Come over to our blog for wholesome recipes and fresh inspiration – **nourishbooks.com.**